HOW TO COPE
SUCCESSFULLY WITH

IRRITABLE BOWEL SYNDROME

RICHARD EMERSON

D1585974

Wellhouse Publishing Ltd

1903784069 01 1C

First published in Great Britain in 2002 by
Wellhouse Publishing Ltd
31 Middle Bourne Lane
Lower Bourne
Farnham
Surrey GU10 3NH

Richard Emerson asserts the moral right to be
identified as the author of this work.

DISCLAIMER

The aim of this book is to provide general information only and should
not be treated as a substitute for the medical advice of your doctor or
any other health care professional. The publisher and author are not
responsible or liable for any diagnosis made by a reader based on the
contents of this book. Always consult your doctor if you are in any way
concerned about your health.

A catalogue record for this book is available from the British Library

ISBN 1 903784 06 9

Printed and bound in Great Britain by
Biddles Ltd., Surrey. www.biddles.co.uk

To Elsie-Louisa Emerson for her love,
support and encouragement

The author would like to thank: Dr Alastair Forbes of St Mark's Hospital; Dr Michael Smyth of Bristol-Myers Squibb; Rhonda Smith of the Digestive Disorders Foundation; Dr Qazim Aziz of Hope Hospital; Megan Tinsdale and Claire Russell of Shire Hall Communications; Sonia Aherne-Conroy; my editor, Barbara Vesey and all at Wellhouse Publishing, for their valuable help, advice and guidance.

Contents

Foreword

In this book Richard Emerson describes Irritable Bowel Syndrome, its nature, causes and management. He has distilled much of what is known scientifically into a nicely balanced volume, and yet without disguising the lack of reliable facts about many aspects of the condition. He illustrates some chapters with an instructive case scenario, and provides a very generous range of treatment options and self-help measures. He acknowledges where these lack support from the medical community, but takes a responsible stance that will make it most unlikely that a sufferer following his suggestions will fall foul of even the most hide-bound, traditional clinician. He has researched his subject remarkably comprehensively and yet manages to keep things brief, to the point and (from my professional perspective) sufficiently intelligible that any interested sufferer should be able to gain many useful hints. I am sure that my own patients will find the book helpful and I will be recommending it strongly.

Alastair Forbes, BSc MD FRCP ILTM,
Consultant Physician and Reader in Gastroenterology,
St Mark's Hospital, London

Introduction

There's only one person who can tackle your irritable bowel symptoms. That person doesn't have a medical practice in Harley Street or a clinic in the Swiss Alps. They're much closer to home than that. He or she is the owner of the face that stares back at you from the bathroom mirror every morning.

You may find that thought hopeful or depressing, but the fact that you're looking at this book suggests you've made a conscious decision to do something. That doesn't mean you're on your own. Your doctor can help and so, I hope, can I. The information within these pages should give you some idea of the nature of irritable bowel syndrome, its causes and - most importantly - its management.

IBS is a common problem, yet the chances are that most of your friends and relatives do not know you have the condition. And it is likely that there are people you know well who have it too, but have concealed that fact from you.

When I was asked to write a book on IBS I thought it would be a project well worth tackling, for several reasons. I knew it was a widespread condition. I had read that it can cause great distress and may severely disrupt people's lives. I also appreciated that many sufferers would rather not talk about it. But as I began to research the topic, what came as a surprise to me was the discovery that I had it, too.

Although I'd been suffering certain symptoms for years, I'd never connected them with IBS. It was not until I began to look into the subject, and in particular to talk to doctors and sufferers, that realization dawned. So writing this book has been a voyage of discovery for me, and I hope reading it will be similarly illuminating for you.

Part One

Understanding IBS

Chapter One

What Is Irritable Bowel Syndrome?

Irritable bowel syndrome (IBS) is a common, painful and often distressing condition suffered by up to one in five of the population at one time or another. In essence it is a problem affecting the body's ability to get rid of waste matter ('faeces' or 'stools').

'Irritable', in this context, means 'abnormally sensitive'. IBS sufferers are sensitive to a whole range of factors, including certain foods. The condition mainly affects the bowel - the lower part of the gastrointestinal tract (or 'gut') - hence the term 'irritable bowel'.

'Syndrome' means there is a distinctive pattern of symptoms. Typically, you have chronic (long-term) constipation or diarrhoea, or find you suddenly switch from one to the other. You also have severe abdominal pain (stomach cramps). Other common symptoms include a feeling of being over-full or bloated, and having severe wind or flatulence. There are less common symptoms as well.

How the Bowel Works

The bowel is the length of gastrointestinal tract that runs between the stomach and the anus. The term 'bowel' includes the small intestine (or small bowel) and the large intestine (or large bowel). To avoid confusion, I am going to use the term 'bowel', rather than 'intestine', from now on.

The small bowel is divided into the duodenum, jejunum and ileum. The large bowel is divided into the caecum, ascending colon, transverse colon, descending colon, sigmoid colon and rectum (see Figure 1).

The latter part of the rectum is known as the anal canal, and ends in two (normally closed) rings of muscle called the internal and external anal sphincters.

Irritable bowel syndrome affects mainly the large bowel and, to a lesser extent, the small bowel.

Bowel Function
The small bowel's job is to complete the breakdown and absorption of food, a process that starts in the mouth and continues in the stomach. The small bowel has special glands that secrete digestive enzymes. These

convert food into molecules small enough to pass through the lining of the small bowel.

At regular intervals throughout the day, a mixture of fluid and food residue (known as chyme) passes into the large bowel. By this stage, the residue is mostly waste. Apart from its water and salt content, it is of little nutritional value.

The large bowel has three tasks - to transport the waste through the body, absorb much (but not all) of its water and salt, and store the remainder until it can be expelled from the body. Semi-dry and dry waste matter is known as stools or faeces. The expulsion of waste is called defaecation.

Figure 1. – The Bowel

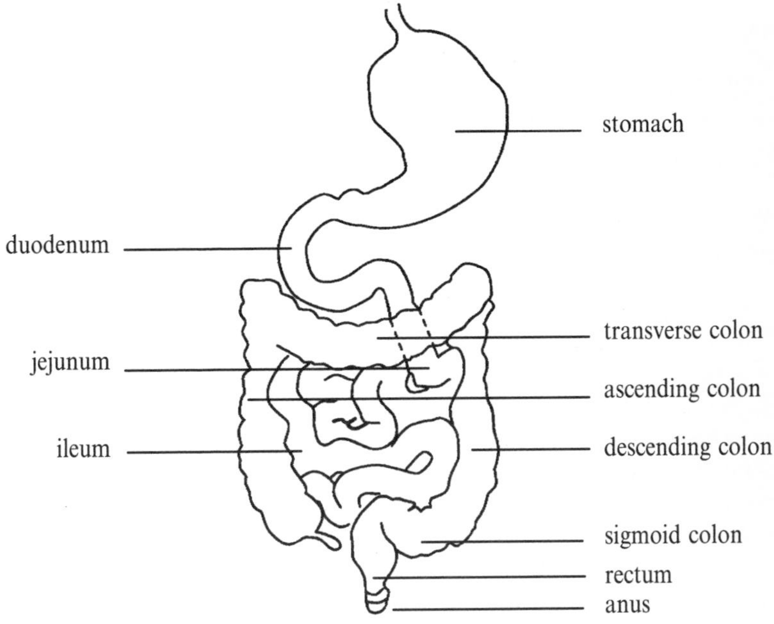

How the Bowel Is Controlled
In order to carry out its various functions, the bowel has several patterns of movement (or motility). The main ones are segmental contractions, which produce a mixing action, and peristalsis, a wave-like squeezing action that pushes food and waste through the bowel - like toothpaste through a tube.

Bowel movement is governed by several control systems involving nerves, hormones and spontaneous electrical activity in the bowel muscles.

The individual cells that make up the smooth muscle inside the bowel wall can contract spontaneously and rhythmically, without receiving any input from the nerves. The job of the various nervous systems linked to the bowel is to control the contractions of the muscle cells so that the muscle layers work in a co-ordinated way, at the appropriate time.

The central nervous system (CNS) is made up of the brain and spinal cord. It is connected to the bowel (and the rest of the gut) via networks of nerves (neurons) and nerve fibres.

One of these networks lies inside the gut and so is termed 'intrinsic'. The gut is the only bodily structure with its own intrinsic nervous system. The others are found outside the gut and are therefore 'extrinsic'.

The intrinsic network is called the enteric system and is responsible for activating the muscles of the gut wall (including the bowel) and activating intestinal mucus production.

The CNS regulates the activity in the bowel by sending signals via the sympathetic and parasympathetic nerves. These two extrinsic networks, in effect, 'pull' in opposite directions. When nerve activity increases in the sympathetic system, the parasympathetic system is damped down, and vice versa. Most of the time the parasympathetic system is the main moderating influence. But during times of stress, sympathetic nerve activity increases, and this affects the bowel.

Food and Stretch Signals

The presence of food (especially a fatty meal) in the stomach is the first trigger for movement in the large bowel. Around three or four times a day, usually after a meal, signals from the stomach cause a wave of contraction known as a mass movement to push faeces through the bowel.

This is the gastrocolic reflex. In effect, the stomach tells the bowel to empty itself to make way for the arrival of more food (and more food waste). The reflex is strongest in the morning, after breakfast (or just a cup of tea or coffee).

In a normal bowel, you are usually only aware of a mass movement when faeces reach the latter part of the bowel - up to 40 minutes after the reflex has occurred. This is why many people get the urge to visit the toilet around 30-40 minutes, on average, after eating food.

Emotional Triggers

Powerful emotions such as aggression, anger, depression, fear, grief, sadness and - of course - stress also influence bowel activity. These emotions affect nervous activity in the sympathetic and parasympathetic nervous systems. This partly explains the link between emotions and the onset of irritable bowel symptoms.

Defaecation Reflex

Waste matter remains in the bowel until a final bowel movement occurs to push faeces out of the body. Defaecation is triggered by the presence of faeces in the final section of bowel, the rectosigmoid (rectum and sigmoid colon).

By the time waste reaches the rectum, it should comprise roughly two parts water to one part solid matter, including undigested plant material, bacteria, bile pigments and a little protein and cholesterol. The stretching sensation caused by the presence of bulky faeces in the rectum triggers the defaecation (or rectocolic) reflex.

In normal circumstances, you can hold back the urge to defaecate until you are able to reach a toilet. Some people can resist this, until the 'need to go' passes. Others find they have only a limited amount of time until the urge is overpowering. These differences are most obvious in IBS sufferers.

Abnormal Bowel Habit

Whether or not your bowel habit is 'abnormal' depends on whether it is causing you distress and affecting your quality of life. People with IBS find that their bowel habit has changed or is inconsistent or excessive, to the point where it is having a serious effect.

You may find you are regular for a while, and then become constipated or suffer diarrhoea, or alternate between the two for no obvious reason. These are, in fact, the three basic conditions seen in IBS so, for convenience, doctors place IBS patients into one of the following categories:

- constipation-predominant IBS (C-IBS),
- diarrhoea-predominant IBS (D-IBS),
- alternating IBS (A-IBS).

In reality it is rarely as straightforward as this. What you may think of as diarrhoea or constipation may differ from your doctor's view. For example, you may believe you have diarrhoea because you go to the toilet up to 10 times a day. Yet on many occasions you may not actually pass a motion. In fact, you might have what you would regard as a 'satisfactory' bowel movement only once or twice a week.

So how do doctors define the three forms of IBS?

Constipation-predominant IBS (C-IBS)

This is defined as having 'difficult or infrequent bowel movements' and is particularly common in women. C-IBS sufferers have difficulty opening their bowels, and little success when straining on the toilet. Any stools may be hard, dry and pellet-like (like rabbit droppings), or pencil- or ribbon-like. They may be accompanied by a white or jelly-like mucus.

Even if sufferers manage to pass a stool, they may not feel completely empty. (This is called a sensation of 'incomplete evacuation'.) They may go to the toilet at the same time each morning, as regular as clockwork then return four or five times during the day because they don't think they have quite finished. People with C-IBS can get preoccupied with their bowels: taking laxatives regularly and spending long periods of time on the toilet - often to little effect.

Diarrhoea-predominant IBS (D-IBS)
This is defined as the 'frequent passing of loose stools' and is more common in men. Typically, D-IBS sufferers visit the toilet several times a day. In many cases, however, the problem is not one of frequency - but urgency. Sufferers may go to the toilet only once or twice a day, which in itself is perfectly normal. But that urge may come on at any time, without warning, and occur with such urgency that sufferers fear they won't get to a toilet in time.

This may lead to occasional bouts of incontinence (or the fear of it) that are both embarrassing and a cause of great anxiety. The fear of the consequences of not reaching the toilet in time can restrict normal life. Sufferers may become reluctant to go out and, in effect, become housebound.

Alternating IBS (A-IBS)
As the name suggests, in this condition sufferers alternate between constipation and diarrhoea. Typically they may have a regular bowel habit for a while, but then suffer constipation. When they next have a bowel movement they may pass a few pellet-like stools followed by loose, watery faeces. The pattern then changes to diarrhoea, and for several days they may be constantly rushing to the toilet until they become regular again. So the cycle is repeated.

Your experience of IBS may be very different from this, however, and your symptoms may not fit conveniently into any of these categories.

Pain and Other Symptoms

All sufferers have abdominal pain. For many people this is the worst aspect of the condition. The pain can vary from mild discomfort to agonizing cramp-like sensations that are so severe you may be doubled up and have to lie down until they ease. The type and degree of pain can vary: it can be described as aching, burning, colicky (that is, coming and going), deep, dull, dragging, griping, nagging, sharp, squeezing and stabbing. The pain may recur regularly over a period of six months or more.

The most common sites of pain are the lower and/or left side of the abdomen, or tucked up under the ribs (called splenic flexure syndrome). It can occur on the right side, low down, or in an unpredictable pattern. Pain may also be felt in other parts of the body, such as the left armpit. The pain may ease after you have a bowel movement, but then return.

You may feel a sharp or stabbing pain in the lower part of the bowel when straining on the toilet (known as proctalgia fugax). Some women have lower abdominal pain, often on the left side, during or after sex.

Bloating and Distension
Another common symptom is abdominal bloating - an unpleasant feeling of fullness, even after small meals. This may prevent you finishing your food. You may also find that your abdomen swells during the day. This may go unnoticed by everyone except you, or may be clearly visible to others. This is known as abdominal distension and can be so apparent that women say they look 'pregnant'.

Characteristically, this is a problem that never occurs at night but starts soon after you wake. Throughout the day your abdomen blows up, becoming more and more uncomfortable. Your clothes get tighter and tighter until your waistband is fully loosened and there are no more buttons left to undo. Your abdomen can feel tender at these times. The distension may disappear if you lie flat on your back or contract your abdominal muscles.

Wind
You may feel full of gas, frequently burping or belching, and have excessive flatulence, perhaps breaking wind embarrassingly in company. The average person releases intestinal gas up to 40 times a day. But in IBS it can happen more often than that. It is not always possible to find somewhere discreet to go to obtain relief so, to avoid embarrassment, sufferers often bottle it up until a convenient moment. The gas build-up can cause pain and nausea, which passes only after sufferers have been able to relieve the pressure by passing wind. (In IBS sufferers, nausea does not usually lead to vomiting.)

Rumbling Stomach
The movement of gas and the semi-liquid contents of the gut, as it shuffles backwards and forwards, poses another problem for IBS sufferers. That is the source of the loud rumbling or gurgling noises (borborygmi) in the abdomen, often heard by others - another source of embarrassment.

Non-bowel Symptoms

You may experience gastrointestinal disorders that are not directly related to the bowel. These include indigestion, lack of appetite or premature satiety - the sensation of feeling full before you have finished a normal-size meal.

There is some overlap between IBS and disorders previously regarded as separate conditions. These include oesophageal reflux (in which stomach contents flow back into the oesophagus - the tube linking the throat and the stomach - causing heartburn) and functional dyspepsia (heartburn, bloating and nausea). Some people alternate between IBS and dyspepsia.

Among IBS sufferers there is a high incidence of 'non-bowel' symptoms, such as muscle and joint pain, headaches, frequent need to urinate, sexual dysfunction (for example, lack of sex drive, inability to achieve or maintain an erection in men, inability to climax in either men or women), disturbed sleep and insomnia, chronic fatigue and tiredness.

Trigger Factors

IBS is usually triggered by certain factors such as stress, emotional upset, anxiety or depression, eating fatty or spicy foods, or drinking alcohol or caffeinated drinks such as tea or coffee.

One person's experience of IBS will be different from another's; not everyone has the same range of symptoms or suffers to the same degree. The onset of symptoms and the severity of an attack can vary, too - not only from person to person, but from day to day and from week to week in the same person. Symptoms can be both persistent and chronic (long term), or disappear for periods of time, only to recur at intervals over the years.

IBS Symptoms

Common symptoms
● Irregular bowel habit
  - constipation (difficult or infrequent bowel movements)
  - diarrhoea (frequent loose stools/urgent need to defaecate)
  - alternating bouts of constipation and diarrhoea
  - urgent need to defaecate but inability to do so
  - sensation of incomplete emptying after defaecating
● Abdominal pain
  - may be intermittent, cramp-like

- may be anywhere in the abdomen, but especially low down, or just under the ribs
- may be relieved by bowel movement and/or passing wind
- stabbing pains in the rectum, especially when straining on the toilet
- bloating, sometimes associated with general abdominal tenderness
- abdominal distension/swelling (often more noticeable on the left side of the abdomen) often associated with tenderness
- gassiness/flatulence/excessive wind
- noisy, rumbling or gurgling sounds emanating from the abdomen
- sense of incomplete evacuation of the bowels
- symptoms aggravated by food and/or stress
- urgent need to open bowels

Less common symptoms
- agitation
- anxiety
- back pain
- depression
- dizziness
- fatigue
- faintness
- weakness
- frequent urination
- headaches
- heartburn/dyspepsia/indigestion
- loss of appetite
- muscle pain
- palpitations
- pain when swallowing (odynophagia), but without food lodging in the throat
- sensation of something stuck in the throat between meals (globus) but without food actually lodging in the throat
- disturbed sleep and/or insomnia

Warning Symptoms
The following are not symptoms of IBS, but may occur along with IBS-like symptoms. They require further investigation and so are known as 'red flags'. See your doctor if you experience:

- bleeding from the anus and/or blood on the faeces (blood on the faeces can be a sign of haemorrhoids, or 'piles' - painfully swollen veins around the anus - which can bleed during defaecation. This is not a

17

'red flag' sign, as such, but should be investigated to rule out other more serious disorders. It also requires treatment in its own right.)

- fever
- weight loss
- persistent, severe indigestion-type pain - especially if it wakes you up at night
- abdominal bloating that persists overnight
- food sticking in the throat (dysphagia)
- vomiting
- breathlessness
- swelling
- rash.

For most people, bowel disorders such as constipation, diarrhoea or wind may be corrected by a change in diet, medication, or simply with time. In IBS sufferers, however, excessive gas, constipation and/or diarrhoea may be the norm, rather than the exception, and there is also the problem of chronic abdominal pain. Clearly, something is wrong with the way the bowel functions in IBS. We'll take a closer look at the causes of this in ChapterThree, but first, in ChapterTwo, we'll discuss who can be affected by IBS.

Case Study: Sonia

Sonia, 25, who works for an ITcompany, has had IBS for several years. Her symptoms began when she was at university: 'Looking back, it was actually just after my mother died when I first got it. I got very constipated and I was taking a laxative two or three times a week just so that I could go to the toilet. But even worse was the terrible stomach cramps and really bad flatulence, which is very embarrassing. It has affected relationships. When you go on a date for the first time you are not sure how he is going to react. Breaking wind is a problem. I've become incredibly 'blokeish' about this and I just make a joke about it. But I know girls who have this problem too, and they just try to hold it in but it can be incredibly painful. The pain eases after you break wind. Another problem is that your stomach really swells up. I've got quite a small waist and it makes me look pregnant. It's worse when I have my period, but that is probably related to the whole stress thing. People do seem to regard IBS as a stress-related illness, and because you get a lot of stress around that time of the month it's going to make it worse.'

Chapter Two

Who Gets IBS?

IBS can affect men and women, young and old. Symptoms can appear at any age, but most often start between the ages of 15 and 25. Some sources say as many as 15 per cent of school-age children may have IBS. The condition can occur periodically throughout life, getting worse, improving or disappearing for a time. The incidence of IBS tends to diminish with age.

Many sufferers don't visit a doctor, however, so no one really knows how widespread the problem is. It is likely that if you are not a sufferer yourself you probably know someone who is (although they may not have told you). Most IBS sufferers cope alone without seeking medical help. Around one in ten have symptoms that are serious enough to require treatment. Typically, they will have had the condition for some months before seeking help. Of those who visit their doctor, one in four will be referred to a hospital specialist for further investigation and treatment.

IBS is the most common condition seen by gastroenterologists (doctors who specialize in digestive disorders), accounting for over half the patients attending out-patient clinics. Of the IBS sufferers who do seek medical help:

- 70 per cent have only mild and infrequent symptoms which do not severely disrupt their lives
- 25 per cent have moderate symptoms that may occasionally interfere with daily activities (missing school, work, or social functions)
- 5 per cent have symptoms that are so severe that their daily activities and quality of life are seriously affected. For them, it is probably of little comfort to know that they are in the minority of IBS sufferers.

IBS is more common among people who have had a very constrained upbringing, or who have been raised outside a normal domestic environment, such as those brought up in institutional care.

Another common factor is physical and/or sexual abuse. In the population as a whole, around one-third of women suffer some form of sexual abuse. But nearly two-thirds of women with IBS have been abused.

IBS is not life-threatening. In fact, most people who are treated for IBS are in good health in all other respects, and usually well-nourished.

Unlike some gastrointestinal disorders, IBS does not prevent absorption of nutrients.

Having said this, IBS symptoms can nevertheless be highly distressing. Around 40 per cent of people with IBS say that it has had a major impact on their lives. At some time they have had to miss work or avoid travelling, socializing, eating certain foods, sex, and domestic and leisure activities. This is because of the pain, or fear of embarrassment of symptoms such as breaking wind, or having a noisy tummy, or often a combination of these.

Those worst affected by IBS may be forced to take more and more time off work, especially when symptoms are severe. In the worst cases, sufferers may limit social engagements or restrict the distances they can travel, for fear of a distressing 'accident' if they can't reach a toilet in time. Some may refuse to leave the house at all, only feeling 'safe' at home.

IBS also affects partners, friends and family. They will be aware of the misery sufferers are going through, but feel powerless to help. They may feel there is little practical help they can give to alleviate the problem, or feel too embarrassed to talk about it or even offer sympathy. When sufferers turn down social invitations for fear of embarrassment or because they are unwell, a partner's social life is affected, too.

Many IBS sufferers may feel that their doctor does not take their symptoms seriously. A misunderstanding can arise when doctors are over-eager to reassure patients that IBS is not life-threatening, like cancer. In doing so, however, the doctor may seem to be dismissing the condition as trivial. If the doctor does not arrange another appointment but simply says, for example, 'Come back and see me if there is no improvement in your symptoms', patients may take this to mean the condition isn't worth treating - or is untreatable. This is not the case.

The Physiology of IBS

IBS is classified as a 'functional bowel disorder'. That is, it is caused by abnormalities in the way the bowel functions. The symptoms of IBS are thought to arise from a combination of the following factors:

- abnormalities in the nervous control of the bowel
- increased sensitivity to internal sensations (stimuli), especially in the bowel, causing the muscular walls of the bowel to spasm
- increased sensitivity or other abnormal reaction to chemicals found in foods, beverages and other substances that triggers symptoms
- the impact on the bowel of certain mental/emotional states, such as anxiety, depression and stress.

Abnormal Nervous Control
In the case of nervous control of the bowel, studies indicate six important differences between sufferers and non-sufferers:

1. The presence of food in the gut has a different effect on those with IBS compared with those not suffering from the syndrome.
2. The bowel's 'pacemaker' cells (interstitial cells of Cajal) are structurally different in IBS sufferers, and cover a smaller area than in non-sufferers. These cells generate slow waves of electrical activity acting like the bowel's own pulse.
3. The frequency of slow-wave (bowel muscle) activity in people with IBS may be as little as half that in non-sufferers.
4. In IBS, the walls of the bowel spasm after only mild stimulation. This seems to be because the bowel is hypersensitive - it shows an exaggerated response to stimuli.
5. Clusters of abnormal muscular contractions occur along the small bowel in IBS sufferers, which may be linked to abdominal cramping and pain.
6. The pressure inside parts of the small bowel (such as the jejunum) is higher than normal.

It is not clear whether all of these differences are significant. But it is likely that some of them are related to the abnormal activity in the bowel wall. In response to stimuli, the bowel muscle contracts in an exaggerated and unco-ordinated (spastic) way.

Painful Spasms
Quite ordinary events, such as eating certain foods, or a build-up of gas, can cause the bowel to over-react, resulting in painful spasms. This disrupts the two main patterns of bowel motility: segmental contraction and peristalsis.

In C-IBS sufferers (and those with A-IBS), the segmental contractions are excessive and unco-ordinated, inhibiting peristalsis and sometimes closing the bowel completely (as well as causing cramping pains). This delays the passage of waste though the bowel, so that the bowel walls absorb most of the water, and the stool becomes compacted - leading to constipation.

In D-IBS sufferers (and, again, those with A-IBS), there are cramping pains and, although peristaltic movements are co-ordinated, they are speeded up. Waste passes through the bowel too quickly, so little water is removed, resulting in loose, watery stools and, hence, diarrhoea.

Chemical Triggers

It is not clear exactly why particular foods trigger symptoms. But it may be that they contain chemicals that cause a particularly intense reaction in chemoreceptors - and other sensors - lining the stomach and bowel.

In a normal subject, chemical signals trigger a wave of contraction that forces waste through the bowel, leading to an urge to defaecate some 30-40 minutes after a meal. But in people with IBS, the signals (or reaction to them) are more marked, causing cramping and - in D-IBS sufferers - more rapid bowel movements.

The strength of the gastrocolic signals emanating from the stomach - and the strength of the bowel's response to them - is partly related to the number of calories in a meal. Fat contains twice the calories of protein (meat and fish) or carbohydrates (bread and potatoes), so fatty foods in the stomach trigger particularly strong muscular contractions.

Any chemical that irritates (or has some other powerfully stimulating effect on) the sensors lining the gut is likely to cause an abnormal reaction. This may explain why substances such as alcohol, nicotine, spicy foods, chocolate and wheat products cause IBS symptoms in some sufferers.

This hypersensitivity is most apparent in the latter part of the bowel, the rectosigmoid, where the presence of faeces results in an almost immediate - and urgent - need to defaecate.

IBS and Stress

You become more aware of the link between your emotional state and your gut at times of heightened emotion. When stressed, tense, anxious, or after a nasty shock, you may get a squeezing sensation in the pit of your stomach. This is caused by increased input from the sympathetic nervous system, which is exerting an effect on normal nerve control in the gut.

This sensation is experienced by everyone, but for those with IBS, stress has a particularly dramatic effect. As with food, a reaction to stress that would be relatively mild in non-sufferers becomes a major reaction in IBS: the bowel goes into spasm, leading to abdominal pain and constipation/diarrhoea.

Even worse, IBS symptoms are highly stressful in themselves, especially if sufferers worry that they have a serious disorder. This leads to a vicious spiral: stress causes symptoms, and the symptoms increase stress levels.

Gas and IBS

It is perhaps not surprising that people with C-IBS should suffer excess flatulence. The longer waste matter remains in the bowel, the more time there is for intestinal bacteria to get to work on it and generate gas.

More surprisingly, perhaps, excess gas is as much - if not more - of a problem in people with D-IBS. The reasons for this are not entirely clear, but it might be that the excessive churning and peristalsis of D-IBS encourages excess gas production. At the same time, the waste passes through the bowel so quickly that little of the gas is absorbed through the lining of the bowel.

Consequently, excess gas builds up and inflates the bowel, causing pain, tenderness, bloating, distension, and chronic flatulence. By expanding the bowel, gas triggers the stretch receptors and so triggers peristalsis and the rectocolic reflex. By voiding gas or faeces, the sufferer gets temporary relief.

Nature or Nurture?

There is still much debate about what causes these underlying differences in IBS symptoms. There is huge variation between different people in terms of looks (body shape and size, for example), personality, and physical and mental abilities. So there is bound to be just as much variation in physiology, such as sensitivity to stimuli arising in the bowel. But does such variation come about by chance - or are other factors at work?

One US study, looking at family dynamics and heredity in IBS, found that patients with IBS were slightly more likely to have children who developed IBS. The reasons for this association are open to debate. Some investigators say it's genetic - the tendency to develop IBS is inherited from our parents.

Others point to factors in childhood environment and/or upbringing - such as inter-family relationships, or learned behaviour. It may be that IBS is due to a combination of all or some of these factors - and others yet unknown.

However, the differences identified in IBS sufferers can also be seen in close relatives who do not have symptoms. This suggests that, although some people may have an inherent weakness that puts them at risk of IBS, whether the symptoms occur depends on other factors, perhaps acting as a kind of 'switch' to set the condition off. One such switch may be a disruption in the balance of bowel micro-organisms, for example, following antibiotic treatment, or severe digestive upset.

The Role of Antibiotics

Many people develop IBS after being given antibiotics. The problem has been noticed especially with tetracyclines, given to treat acne, and following pelvic surgery (such as hysterectomy), when antibiotics are routinely used to prevent infection.

Antibiotics not only destroy the pathogenic bacteria they are aimed at, but also the beneficial bacteria in the bowel. Harmful organisms such as the yeast infection *Candida albicans*, and disease-causing bacteria such as *Escherichia coli*, *Staphylococcus* and *Campylobacter*, are kept in check by the presence of these friendly microbes.

Fungal microbes, however, are not affected by antibiotics. And pathogenic bacteria are often more resistant to antibiotics than are 'native' bacteria, so their numbers recover more quickly after drug treatment is stopped.

Whatever the reason, this leaves the path clear for a massive expansion in fungal and bacterial pathogens. These microbes then release toxins which irritate and 'sensitize' the bowel, so triggering the development of IBS.

Many people with IBS date the onset of the condition to severe digestive upset, such as gastroenteritis - often due to food poisoning contracted while on holiday abroad. This may be because (as with antibiotic treatment) the large numbers of pathogenic bacteria irritate the bowel lining, causing hypersensitivity to all stimuli.

The Psychological Switch

Not everyone traces IBS symptoms to antibiotics or infection, however. Studies on IBS patients have revealed a high incidence of psychological factors such as:

- major trauma - accidental injury; violent physical or sexual assault; long-term emotional, physical or sexual abuse; witnessing a traumatic event
- institutional care - being raised in a children's home, or by foster parents; educated at boarding school or academy; time in a detention centre
- psychological illness - chronic anxiety states; panic disorder; obsessive-compulsive disorder; severe depression
- major life event - bereavement; moving house; changing or losing jobs.

While IBS is definitely not 'all in the mind', this shows that the mind - or at least the brain - plays a significant part in IBS.

Researchers are studying this brain - bowel link to try to explain:

- why IBS sufferers are hypersensitive to sensations others do not notice
- why these sensations cause such an extreme reaction in IBS sufferers, when they trigger a normal response, or none at all, in others.

Current lines of research point to differences in the way that IBS sufferers register pain, and how signals from the bowel are processed in the brain and perceived as painful. These are the subjects of Chapter Three.

There is still no drug or other treatment that can 'cure' IBS, but this doesn't mean the outlook for sufferers is gloomy. In many cases the condition clears up of its own accord, often relatively quickly.

Even in persistent cases, there is much that can be done to control symptoms. Most chronic sufferers learn to manage IBS through a combination of simple lifestyle changes, self-help measures, over-the-counter remedies and, where appropriate, prescription drugs and/or therapy. Many people manage to alleviate their symptoms completely by this means.

Others find that by managing the condition they can lessen their symptoms to the extent that IBS causes only minimal disruption to their lives. They say they no longer feel preoccupied with - or dominated by - the condition and so can lead full, active, 'normal' lives.

Case Study: Alan

Alan is an engineer working for a medical equipment company: 'I tried all the over-the-counter remedies, but the symptoms just came on so quickly. I missed so many days at work that my job was at risk. I was too embarrassed to tell my boss the real reason I was always out of the office. I used up virtually all of last year's leave as sick days. But since I've been seeing a doctor I have been doing a lot better. The doctor gave me some medication [an antispasmodic] and that helps sometimes, although not always. But I still have some of the old symptoms. The doctor said I should spend more time on myself, just relaxing and taking it easy, and doing deep breathing exercises and that sort of thing. He told me that although stress is not the cause of my condition it probably aggravates it. Actually, I think I began to feel a lot better when the doctor said what my problem was and that it wasn't anything more serious - cancer or something. That really put my mind at rest. I'm thinking of doing something like yoga that is supposed to be good for relaxing you.'

Chapter Three

What Causes the Pain of IBS?

Studies suggests that the pain, and other symptoms, of IBS may be related to abnormalities in the 'brain-gut axis' - the nerve pathways between the bowel and the brain. To see how these pathways work, we need to look at the nature of pain itself.

What Is Pain?

There are countless sensors (receptors) all over the body, both inside and out, that detect, for example, touch, temperature, movement and pressure. It's natural, therefore, to think that the body is equipped with 'pain sensors' too. This assumes that pain is something 'out there' - like heat, movement and pressure - that we come into contact with.

But pain is more complicated than this, as the mysterious phenomenon of phantom limb pain (PLP) demonstrates. PLP sufferers feel pain in an arm or a leg that they have lost, for example, through accident or surgery - they would have lost the limb's 'pain sensors' at the same time.

Nociceptors and Reflexes

In fact, instead of pain sensors, we have free nerve endings called *nociceptors* (pronounced 'no-see-septors'), on sensory neurons. Nociceptors detect 'noxious' or unpleasant stimuli, such as damage caused to the tissues.

When you prick your finger on a thorn or tread on a pin, the damaged cells release histamine. This chemical activates nearby nociceptors, which send signals along their nerve fibres to the spinal cord. Here, they activate motor neurons that control muscles in the limb. The motor neurons activate the muscles, which jerk the limb out of harm's way. This is a reflex action.

In the spinal cord nociceptive neurons also connect with nerve cells, called transmission neurons, which send information about the tissue damage to the brain. The brain processes the signals to give our conscious perception of pain. The purpose of registering pain, in this case, is to encourage you to get the wound treated and make sure you learn from the experience - so you take more care in the future!

A and C Fibres

There are two kinds of nerve that carry messages from the nociceptors to the spinal cord - fast A-fibres, and slower C-fibres. The signals that travel along the A-fibres give the initial sensation of pain - one that is sharp, localized and distinct. The signals that travel along the slower C-fibres produce a more persistent sensation - one of a dull and more generalized pain.

The Healing Power of Rubbing

Signals from nociceptors do not always register as pain, however. They can be blocked by signals from other types of sensor - such as mechanoreceptors, which detect touch, pressure and movement, and thermoreceptors, which detect heat and cold.

These sensors are connected to interneurons which, in turn, connect with transmission neurons in the spinal cord. When activated, signals from the mechanoreceptors and thermoreceptors block the nociceptor signals. This is part of an anti-pain mechanism called the 'pain gate' (see Figure 2).

Figure 2. – The Pain Gate

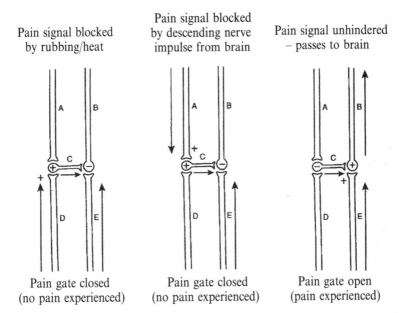

Pain signal blocked
by rubbing/heat

Pain signal blocked
by descending nerve
impulse from brain

Pain signal unhindered
– passes to brain

Pain gate closed
(no pain experienced)

Pain gate closed
(no pain experienced)

Pain gate open
(pain experienced)

Key:
A – descending anti-pain pathway
B – ascending pain pathway
C – interneuron ("pain gate")

D – thick sensory fibre
E – thin nociceptor ("pain sensor") fibre

You have probably activated the pain gate yourself, for example by rubbing a bruised knee or applying a cold compress to a swollen ankle. This anti-pain effect is one reason why touch therapies, such as massage, or hot and cold compresses used in hydrotherapy, can offer pain-relief.

Mind Over Pain

Other nerve fibres link up with the pain gate, too. These are called 'descending pathways' and originate from parts of the brain known as the anti-nociceptive pain modulating system (APMS).

When activated, signals travel down the descending pathways to the level where the nociceptor signals enter the spinal cord. The descending signals trigger release of pain killing chemicals (such as endorphins, enkephalins and dynorphins), which close the pain gate and block the nociceptor signals.

If the nociceptor signals increase, the brain responds with a more powerful blocking signal. Many low-frequency signals from nociceptors are blocked by the APMS automatically - without you noticing them.

Signals from nociceptors only register as pain when they reach a certain threshold. You can block the pain gate artificially with painkilling drugs, such as morphine (which are chemically similar to endorphins). But it is possible to activate the anti-pain pathways in other ways. This may be the way hypnosis blocks pain. On the other hand, certain drugs, including caffeine, interfere with the APMS and make pain worse.

Somatic and Visceral Pain

IBS sufferers can cope well with 'external pain' stimuli in which subjects can see the painful stimulus (also called somatic pain). In experiments in which subjects had to keep their hands in a bucket of icy water for as long as possible, people with IBS could tolerate the cold better than others. But IBS sufferers are much more sensitive to internal pain (or visceral pain), affecting the bowel and other internal organs.

Visceral Signals

Much of the time we are unaware of gut sensations. Sometimes, signals from the abdomen make us aware of hunger, fullness or, occasionally, mild digestive upset. More unpleasant stimuli may be experienced as pain. A feeling of rectal 'fullness' is felt as an urgent need to evacuate your bowels. This can become increasingly painful if there is no toilet handy. A gastrointestinal upset may cause abdominal cramping or colicky pain.

We are aware of these stimuli because of sensors in the gut. These send signals along sensory nerve fibres to the spinal cord and thence to the brain for processing. As mentioned, there are several types of gut sensor:

- nociceptors - which detect, for example, inflammation
- chemoreceptors - which detect hormones and other chemicals
- thermoreceptors - which detect temperature changes and respond to, for example, a hot or cold drink
- low- and high-threshold mechanoreceptors - which react to stretching, for example, as bulky food or food waste passes along the gut.

Low-threshold sensors register normal pressures, and high-threshold sensors respond to high pressures and distention. High-threshold sensors may be as important as nociceptors for the symptoms of pain in IBS.

PainTest

Gut sensations are the same whether or not you have IBS, yet IBS sufferers are more likely to perceive such stimuli as painful. This has been demonstrated in experiments involving a barostat balloon.

When this balloon was inserted into the rectum of IBS sufferers and non-sufferers and slowly inflated, subjects were asked to report when they first experienced pain. Few of the non-IBS sufferers reported any pain - even when the balloon was inflated to its maximum volume of 180 mls.

Some IBS subjects reported discomfort or pain when the balloon was only partially inflated, and more than 50 per cent complained of acute pain when the balloon was inflated to 180 mls. This shows that IBS subjects perceive bowel sensations more intensely than do non-sufferers, and are aware of them for longer. In a second test, experimenters introduced a painful stimulus into the sigmoid colon of IBS sufferers. The nerves supplying this region of the bowel are distinct from those supplying the rectum. Yet when this test was followed by a repeat of the balloon experiment, even those IBS sufferers who could previously tolerate the barostat balloon now reported pain.

This shows that, in IBS sufferers, a painful stimulus in one part of the bowel leads to hyperalgesia (increased pain-sensitivity) in another part. This may be because of the way nerve fibres transmit stimuli from the bowel.

PainThreshold in IBS

There are three main types of transmission nerve fibre responsible for carrying nerve signals from the bowel up the spinal cord to the brain. These are low-threshold (L) fibres, high-threshold (H) fibres, and mechanically insensitive (MI) fibres. These fibres are linked to nociceptive neurons in the bowel and also to regulatory neurons, which send information regulating movement and secretion in the bowel (and other parts of the gut).

Most bowel sensations are low key and trigger only L-fibres, which activate regulatory neurons, not nociceptive neurons. But a stronger signal activates the H-fibres, and increases signal traffic along the pain pathways. Once processed in the brain, these signals may be perceived as pain. These sensations are usually short-lived and the system soon returns to normal.

However, if a stimulus arising from the general region of the bowel is particularly intense, frequently repeated or long-lasting, for example due to severe inflammation or physical injury, all three types of fibre are activated, including the MI-fibres. This, in turn, lowers the threshold throughout the pain system, including neurons and nerve fibres connected to the nearby region of the spinal cord.

In due course, threshold levels return to normal in some parts of the nerve network, but stay low in the spinal cord. As a result, sensations that before would only have triggered L-fibres now activate pain pathways, leading to hypersensitivity in the bowel.

In non-IBS sufferers the pain threshold returns to its normal setting within a short time. But in people with IBS, this hypersensitivity lasts much longer. Signals from the bowel become amplified and the threshold for reacting to them becomes lowered.

The tendency to develop this sensitivity may be related to an innate structural weakness in the bowel. But there must also be a physical or psychological 'switch' that is so severe it triggers the development of IBS symptoms.

These 'switches' (antibiotics, infection, surgery and physical or sexual abuse, as already mentioned) may be repeated, prolonged or intense enough to lower the threshold for pain for hours, days or even longer.

IBS sufferers then continue to be aware of all sensations in the bowel (even innocuous ones). The arrival of certain foodstuffs or the passage of bulky faeces that would normally be unnoticed or cause minimal reaction in a non-IBS person, causes an abnormal reaction in people with IBS.

The bowel wall goes into spasm, causing unco-ordinated and/or increased bowel movements. Pain pathways are activated and the information is processed in the brain to give our conscious perception of pain.

Referred Pain

Some nerve pathways from the bowel converge with other pathways arising from different parts of the body. This can give a false location for the pain - a condition known as referred pain. This may be why IBS symptoms can include parts of the body unconnected with the gut, such as the armpit.

While all this helps to explain why IBS sufferers are hypersensitive to bowel sensations, it does not explain why psychological factors play such an important part, nor why symptoms come and go. This relates to the psychology of pain.

What Part Does the Mind Play in IBS?

The perception of pain is not just an automatic reaction to a set of signals. The brain must first process this information and formulate a response.

How the Brain Processes Pain

Pain-processing in the brain is made up of three elements: discrimination, evaluation, and emotion. The way these elements interact, and the relative contribution each one makes, determine whether or not bowel (and other) sensations are perceived as painful and, if so, the level of that pain.

- Discrimination occurs in the outer brain (somatosensory cortex). This identifies, for example, where the sensation is coming from.
- Evaluation takes place at the front of the brain (prefrontal lobes). This determines the severity (severe or minor) and quality (stabbing or aching, for example) of the sensation.
- Emotional response occurs in the mid-brain (limbic system). This creates feelings such as being 'wracked', 'tortured' or 'nauseated'.

A Unique Experience

Your psychological profile also plays an important part in this. Everyone is different - physically, mentally and emotionally. Your home environment, upbringing, relationships and personal history are unique to you. So the way you respond to unpleasant sensations (whether they are perceived as painful and, if so, how painful) is unique, too.

The experience of pain differs not only from person to person but also from time to time in the same person, depending on factors such as your sleep-wake cycle and hormone levels. For example, we are most sensitive to pain between midnight and 4 a.m., and least sensitive between 4 p.m. and 7 p.m.

Also important are your hormone levels (especially a woman's menstrual cycle), stress levels and emotional state at a given time. For example, anticipating pain (a dental appointment, perhaps) can intensify pain. Excitement, on the other hand, whether on a sports field or a battle field, can reduce, or even suppress, pain.

Pain is also determined by heredity (genetic makeup) and whether you have been brought up to feel you shouldn't 'make a fuss' (upbringing).

Another factor is the number of stressful events (stressors) you have experienced, and how you have learned to cope with them. These might include 'life factors' such as poor housing conditions and troubled relationships, or traumatic events such as chronic and/or life-threatening illness, injury, or physical or sexual abuse.

The Emotional Motor System

Pain-processing is co-ordinated by a network of structures within the limbic system called the emotional motor system (EMS). The EMS processes the data from the somatosensory cortex (discrimination), the prefrontal lobes (evaluation), the rest of the limbic system (emotional response) and, via the spinal cord, from the internal organs (including bowel sensations).

The EMS also records your physiological state (hormone levels), mental/emotional state (anxiety, depression, stress) and takes into account previous experience of similar sensations (memory), and how you have learned to respond to such sensations (conditioning).

The EMS then sends out signals to suppress or accentuate various control systems. For example, the EMS can activate the sympathetic nervous system. This affects bowel movements and leads to the release of histamine and seratonin (chemicals also associated with inflammation), causing hyperalgesia (increased pain-sensitivity) and muscle spasms.

The EMS also affects pain pathways, intensifying signals from the bowel, inhibiting anti-pain pathways which would normally suppress low-key signals from the bowel, and increasing pain perception. As a result, you are more aware of bowel sensations, and more likely to perceive them as painful.

The EMS's influence on the autonomic nervous system has wide-ranging effects throughout the body. This may explain why IBS can cause such varied symptoms, including indigestion, urinary problems, muscle pains and sexual dysfunction - all systems under autonomic control.

The involvement of the EMS may also help to explain why the tendency to develop IBS arises through a complex interplay of physiological and psychological factors including genetic makeup, upbringing, traumas and other stressors - and especially a combination of such factors - during life.

As your emotional and physical state changes over days, weeks and months, there is a characteristic increase or decrease in symptoms - or even a remission - until the cycle begins again.

Although the EMS (and its effect on the autonomic nervous system) is not under conscious control, never underestimate the capacity of the conscious mind to influence it - as the 'placebo effect' proves.

Placebo Effect

A placebo is a dummy pill (traditionally a sugar pill) used as a control when testing a new drug. In theory, if patients treated with the test drug get better while those taking the placebo do not, the new drug must work. Except it doesn't always work out that way. Often, people taking the placebo get better too. This is the placebo effect.

To get the placebo effect, you must be convinced that the placebo drug is genuine and have confidence in the doctor, nurse or therapist who is administering it. This effect doesn't only work with drugs. A bogus therapy can also have a placebo effect, so long as patients have confidence in it.

Faith in the therapy may affect pain-processing and, via the EMS, activate descending 'anti-pain' pathways. Acting through the autonomic nerves, the EMS may also lower blood pressure, moderate bowel activity and have other beneficial effects.

The very fact that a doctor, nurse or therapist takes an interest may reduce your stress and anxiety levels which (via the EMS) can alter your perception of pain. Many forms of orthodox and complementary therapy may work, in part, by tapping into these unconscious processes.

Similarly self-help techniques such as positive thinking, meditation, and visualization; and psychological therapies such as counselling, may involve such unconscious brain-gut connections. These subjects are covered in Parts 2 and 3.

Case Study: Julia

Julia, 29, is a freelance illustrator who dates her symptoms to a stomach bug she picked up while on holiday in Mexico: 'I get very constipated, but then sometimes when I eat something I have to rush to the toilet. But then I can't go! It's so frustrating! The pain has been bad at times but I think the worst thing is the bloating and wind. It's ruined my sex life. Men think it's really funny when they, you know, break wind. But they don't think it is so funny when I do it. It can happen at any time, even during sex. I've stopped dating now. My last boyfriend thought I was mad because I kept running up to the bathroom. But unless I get rid of the wind the pain is unbearable. The more anxious I get the worse it gets.'

Chapter Four

Should You See a Doctor?

Many people with IBS put off seeing their doctor for a long time. Often they don't want to bother the doctor over 'something trivial'. Sometimes they are worried they've got something life-threatening.

You should never suffer in silence like this, or worry needlessly. If you aren't sure whether you need to visit your doctor, ask yourself the following questions:

- Have you been suffering IBS symptoms for more than a few weeks?
- Have you tried the standard over-the-counter remedies without success?
- Are the symptoms serious enough to affect your quality of life?
- Are you worried about your health?

If the answer to any of these is yes, you should seriously consider consulting your doctor.

How the Doctor Can Help
While there is no test that can confirm or rule out IBS, your doctor will probably be able to diagnose IBS simply on the basis of your symptoms, and possibly after a physical examination, especially if you are under 40.

In some cases the doctor may want to carry out more tests or refer you to a specialist for further investigation. This is to rule out other conditions that can cause IBS-like symptoms. If your have IBS, these tests usually draw a blank. Of course, the doctor may find that you have another similar disorder - apart from IBS - but this is not very common.

There are many disorders that cause symptoms similar to those of IBS. They include inflammatory bowel diseases (such as Crohn's disease or ulcerative colitis), bowel cancer, cancer of the rectum, certain disorders involving the thyroid gland, and even parasitic infestations.

Special tests are warranted mainly in older people, or patients whose symptoms do not quite match the standard pattern for IBS, or those with a medical or family history of digestive disorders. Of most concern are those with non-IBS symptoms - so-called 'alarm' or 'red flag' symptoms, such as blood in the stools, unexplained weight loss, vomiting, breathlessness, swelling or a rash.

Preparing for the Consultation

Before you go to the doctor, it might help if you make notes about your symptoms. You can then answer the doctor's questions in enough detail to enable him or her to reach a confident diagnosis. Think about the best way to describe your symptoms, especially pain:

● What can you compare the pain with, to help the doctor understand? For example, is it a burning pain, or more like a dull ache?
● Where do you usually feel this pain - in the upper abdomen, just under your ribcage, lower down, to one side, or all over the abdominal area?
● How often do you have symptoms (every month, every day, more than once a day) and at what time of day (morning, afternoon, evening)?
● Have you noticed if certain factors (foods, stress, start of your period) seem to bring on symptoms?

Note Down What the Doctor Says

Remember to take your notes with you to the doctor. It's a good idea to take a notepad and pen along too, so you can write down what the doctor says. Don't be afraid to ask the doctor to repeat information or explain anything you don't understand. You might even take a tape-recorder and record the consultation. As a matter of courtesy, ask the doctor if he or she objects to this. Doctors don't usually mind. They realize it can be hard for patients to take in everything they are told, especially when nervous.

The Consultation

The doctor will ask about your symptoms, their severity and frequency. Try to give as much information as possible. Details of your bowel habit will be especially important if the doctor is to diagnose IBS. You may find the topic embarrassing, but rest assured your doctor has discussed the subject many times before and will not feel at all awkward.

Your doctor will ask whether you ever have symptoms at night. Unlike some other gastrointestinal disorders, IBS symptoms usually occur only when you are awake. Nocturnal symptoms suggest a different condition.

Medical History

Many people date the onset of IBS to a single event, such as an accident, illness or medical treatment. So you will be asked about your medical history - that is, whether you have had any diseases in the past that might have a bearing on your condition. For example, have you had food poisoning - especially while on holiday? Mention whether you have had an operation (not only involving the abdomen) or have taken a course of antibiotics.

The doctor will also ask you about your family's medical history. For example, whether a parent, sibling or other close relative has had bowel cancer, as a susceptibility to this disease may run in families.

You should mention other factors that might be relevant. For example, say whether you feel anxious, depressed or stressed at the moment. Your emotional state can trigger IBS, and this information helps the doctor reach a diagnosis. The doctor will probably ask you about your diet, as foods can also be a significant aspect. If you are taking medicines or food supplements of any kind, take them along to show the doctor.

Rome Criteria

In order to reach a diagnosis of IBS, your doctor may follow certain guidelines. The best known (and still widely used) are the Manning criteria, first published in the 1970s. These are being replaced by the more recent 'Rome criteria', first published in 1989, which were revised and simplified in 1999 as 'Rome II'.

The Rome criteria were developed by multinational teams that reviewed all the studies on IBS to produce these guidelines:

● Symptoms must be present for at least 12 weeks or more in the previous 12 months (this can apply to any 12 weeks in a year, so symptoms need not be consecutive)
● There is abdominal discomfort or pain that has two of the following three features -
   1. the abdominal discomfort or pain is relieved with defaecation
   2. the onset of abdominal discomfort or pain is associated with a change in frequency of stool
   3. the onset of abdominal discomfort or pain is associated with a change in the appearance of stool.

According to the Rome criteria, the doctor can be even more confident of a diagnosis of IBS if the patient reports any of the following symptoms:

● abnormal stool frequency - more than three bowel movements per day or fewer than three per week
● abnormal stool form - stools are lumpy or hard or loose or watery - in more than one out of four defaecations
● abnormal stool passage - straining, urgency, or feeling of incomplete evacuation - in more than one out of four defaecations
● passage of mucus in more than one out of four defaecations
● bloating or abdominal distension on more than one out of four days
● absence of any physical/biochemical abnormalities that might explain the symptoms.

Physical Examination

Your doctor may carry out a physical examination, especially of the abdomen, to check for pain or tenderness, lumps, swellings, hard or compacted areas, or signs of growths or obstructions that might suggest other conditions or (if absent) help to confirm IBS. The examination may reveal surgical scars - indicating the site of past abdominal surgery. The doctor may hear rumbling noises coming from your tummy.

If you have IBS, you may notice some tenderness if the doctor presses down on the left side of your abdomen (over the sigmoid colon), or just below the ribs. If you are very constipated, the bowel may feel slightly firm.

In some cases, the doctor may carry out a digital rectal examination. Here the doctor inserts a rubber-gloved finger into your anus.

Management Regime

If the doctor diagnoses IBS he or she may prescribe medication, such as a laxative, an antidiarrhoeal or an antispasmodic. But many doctors prefer to delay giving medication until you have followed a simple management regime, involving basic lifestyle measures.

You might be asked to keep an IBS diary (see Chapter Five), change your diet (Chapters Six and Seven), manage your stress (Chapter Eight) and pain (Chapter Nine). The surgery may organize stress- or pain-management classes you can attend. And you may be asked to plan a diet with a dietitian.

You'll probably be asked to come back in a few weeks so that the doctor can assess your progress. Any reduction in your symptoms in the meantime will help to confirm the doctor's initial diagnosis.

Reassurance

The doctor will reassure you that irritable bowel is not a life-threatening condition, will not progress to a more serious condition, and that surgery will not be necessary. You will also be told that, in most cases, the condition resolves by itself in time. In saying this your doctor is not trivializing your symptoms, or suggesting that they are imaginary. He or she is simply trying to put your mind at rest by ruling out other conditions. This can also help to reduce any anxiety that may be exacerbating your symptoms.

Your doctor realizes that IBS is a distressing condition and will want to do everything possible to help you. If, however, you feel the doctor is not taking your symptoms seriously enough, you are entitled to ask for another doctor's opinion or seek referral to a specialist.

Diagnostic Tests

Your doctor may decide to carry out additional tests if he or she is not completely satisfied that you have IBS. Family doctors can arrange basic tests themselves. For more sophisticated tests, the doctor may refer you to a gastroenterologist, based at a local hospital.

Blood Tests

The doctor may take a sample of blood for laboratory examination. This is to check your:

- blood count - the number of red blood cells (erythrocytes) present (this can identify some forms of anaemia)
- erythrocyte sedimentation rate - the rate at which the red blood cells settle out in a test tube (this checks for neoplastic disease - abnormal cell growth that may develop into cancer - or inflammatory disorders)
- serum chemistries - to evaluate liver and kidney function.

Stool Tests

You may be asked to provide a stool sample, which will be examined in a laboratory. One is known as a faecal occult blood test (in medical terminology, occult means 'hidden'). This test is carried out to look for traces of hidden blood that are too small to spot visually (possibly revealing inflammatory bowel disorders or cancer).

Laboratory staff will also evaluate the colour and consistency of the stool, and will test for bacteria, parasitic worms and their eggs, and parasitic amoeba (or other single-celled animals) and their cysts (to check for infection/infestation). In some cases, staff may test for traces of fats (indicating poor absorption of nutrients).

Endoscopic Examination

The doctor may arrange for an endoscopic examination, which is usually carried out in a hospital. In this procedure the doctor examines the inside of the bowel using an endoscope - a long, flexible, illuminated viewing tube - that is gently inserted via the anus.

An endoscopic examination of the latter part of the bowel (the sigmoid colon) is called sigmoidoscopy, and only needs a relatively short, and often rigid, device. An endoscopic examination of other parts of the bowel is called colonoscopy, and requires a longer and more flexible instrument.

The doctor looks for abnormal signs such as inflammation or ulceration which would indicate an inflammatory disease such as ulcerative colitis. Endoscopes are usually equipped with miniature tools that enable the operator to remove a small portion of tissue so it can be examined in a laboratory. This is called a biopsy.

Preparing for Endoscopy

You will need to take laxatives and fast for a day before the examination. Endoscopy is not usually painful but can cause unpleasant internal sensations and some discomfort. As part of the procedure, air or gas may be blown into the bowel to expand it (a process known as insufflation). This is done to make the bowel easier to inspect visually, but some IBS sufferers may find this causes a painful stretching sensation.

You may be given sedatives, a local anaesthetic (to numb the anal area) and drugs to dry up internal secretions. Afterwards you may have wind pains and flatulence for a short time, and may feel rather dehydrated. If a biopsy is carried out, you may notice traces of blood in your stool. If you notice more than a trace, contact your doctor at once.

Barium X-ray

Your doctor may arrange for a barium enema X-ray. In this procedure a rubber tube is gently inserted into the anus and then a liquid substance such as barium sulphate is poured into the tube. This will enable the radiographer to get a clear X-ray photograph of the bowel. (Barium is a metal element that is opaque to X-rays.)

The procedure lasts for about half an hour and, although tiring, usually causes only mild discomfort. Most of the barium passes out of the anus soon afterwards, and the rest is excreted later. To highlight other areas of the digestive tract, barium sulphate may be administered as a 'meal' (actually a drink), or a 'swallow' (a thick paste).

Scans

The doctor may carry out other investigations such as:
- ultrasound - ultrasonic sound waves that give an image of the bowel
- computed tomography (CT) scan - computer-enhanced X-rays that produce highly detailed images of the bowel.

Other Tests

Other tests may be considered if the patient's medical or family history or other factors seem to warrant them. They include the following - mainly to discover possible causes of chronic diarrhoea:
- lactose breath hydrogen test, to check for lactose intolerance (an inability to digest lactose, a form of sugar found in milk)
- thyroid-stimulating hormone determination, to check for an overactive thyroid gland

- glucose tolerance, to test for diabetes
- coeliac sprue serology, to check for coeliac disease (adverse reaction to gluten, a protein found in wheat products).

If any tests reveal disorders other than (or in addition to) IBS, the doctor will prescribe the appropriate treatment. For IBS itself, a management regime is the next step. This is dealt with in Part 2.

Case Study: John
John, 47, is the financial director for a large retail chain. He says: 'I'd had a problem for years before I went to my doctor. He told me he thought it was irritable bowel syndrome. I didn't realize there would be a proper name for it. I just called it my 'tummy trouble'. I get a certain amount of pain and some flatulence. But the main problem is the diarrhoea. It's not that I have to go to the toilet that often. But it comes on without warning and the urge is so strong I'm worried I won't make it in time. To get to my office is a 10 mile journey across the city. I have to do that twice a day, usually in heavy traffic. It would have been stressful anyway, but because of my irritable bowel problem, when I need to go I really need to go. So I have had to learn where every toilet is on my route. I don't just mean public toilets, but every petrol station that has a toilet, every shop where I can stop and knock on the door and know they'll let me use their toilet, and every pub that is open at the times when I'm driving past.'

Part Two
Managing IBS

Chapter Five

Lifestyle

There is no 'magic pill' or other treatment currently available that offers a complete solution to IBS. The best approach is to manage the condition by means of self-help measures and lifestyle changes - plus medication, if necessary (see Chapter Nine). The aim is to make that psychological leap from being an 'IBS sufferer' to someone who has IBS but is coping with it.

If the symptoms are relatively mild and the attacks infrequent, self-help measures may be sufficient. Always bear in mind that, even in the worst cases, symptoms often clear up of their own accord (known as spontaneous remission) regardless of any measures or medication you may take.

A Multi-directional Approach

As IBS is such a complex condition arising from the way the brain and bowel interact, it follows that you will need to tackle the condition from several directions. By identifying factors that seem to trigger an attack, you should find the right combination of measures to control the condition. Once the physical symptoms of IBS are no longer ruling your life, your mental and physical well-being may improve dramatically too.

Keeping an IBS Diary

You should keep an IBS diary to record your symptoms and factors that trigger them. One way is to use a large-format diary or notebook and divide the pages into sections. In one section record your daily symptoms, such as the frequency of your visits to the toilet, the degree of abdominal pain and bloating, and any other, less-common symptoms, such as nausea and headaches. Use a scale of one to ten to indicate the severity of the pain.

In the other sections, write down any potential triggers. Be sure to note any factors that might be relevant, whether or not there is an obvious connection. Categories you might consider include:
- food - including snacks
- drinks - hot beverages and fizzy drinks
- cigarettes, alcohol - and other recreational drugs
- emotional state - whether happy, relaxed, anxious or depressed
- general health - not only disorders such as colds and flu but whether you are tired or rundown

- stressors - such as a heavy workload, tight deadlines, rows (and other relationship problems), travel (including holidays) and menstrual cycle
- medication - both prescription drugs and over-the-counter remedies. (Some medicines, especially ones given for high blood pressure and anxiety, can cause symptoms such as constipation.)

Look for a Pattern
Every week, highlight which factors crop up regularly in association with certain symptoms. After a while you should see a pattern. For example, you might notice that a fatty meal seems to trigger diarrhoea and abdominal pain, especially when you are overworked or have had a row.

Look at Your Lifestyle

Your IBS symptoms may well be the incentive you've been waiting for to make some radical and long-overdue changes to your lifestyle. Now is the time to consider which areas are in need of improvement.

Changing Your Eating Pattern
The first step is to look at your diet and eating habits. Quite often it is not only foods that cause a problem, but the way or amount you eat. Bolting your food or eating big meals can quickly overload - and overstretch - the bowel, triggering spasms and leading to cramping and/or diarrhoea. Eating at irregular times and constant snacking - especially of high-sugar, high-fat foods - can also cause symptoms.

Allow yourself plenty of time to eat. Think of mealtimes as an enjoyable break in the day - not a waste of valuable time. Plan tasty meals so you look forward to your food. Chew slowly and pause between mouthfuls to give the food time to go down. Allow time between courses, and more time afterwards to sit and relax.

You may find you suffer fewer symptoms if you have regular mealtimes, eat smaller meals, or smaller portions, and have healthy snacks such as fruit between meals if you get hungry. The old rule that 'you should leave the table wanting more' makes a lot of sense for IBS sufferers. (Which foods to eat and which ones to avoid are covered in the next two chapters.)

Things to Do

There are other measures you can try to manage your symptoms. These include psychological ones, such as adopting a positive outlook, and practical ones, such as taking regular exercise. These simple steps can also go a long way to improving your general health and mental well-being.

Think Positive

Studies involving psychological profiling techniques indicate a strong link between IBS symptoms and mental outlook. A high percentage of IBS patients seem to take a pessimistic view of life and feel they have only limited control over what happens to them (see ChapterTen).

But the link between your conscious thoughts and your mental/emotional state works both ways. Just as being depressed, say, can give you a rather negative outlook, so adopting a positive outlook can lift your depression.

Positive Affirmations

One approach is through the technique of *positive affirmations*. These are statements you make to enforce a positive outlook and counteract negative feelings. You should recite your affirmations several times a day. Find a method that suits you. For example, each morning stand in front of your mirror and make a positive statement such as:

- 'I feel strong and confident. I can handle whatever the day may bring.'
- 'I feel happy, contented and at peace with the world.'
- 'I recognize the good and the valuable in myself and in everyone I meet.'

You can adapt these affirmations, or make up your own. Choose a sentiment that is appropriate to your personality and aspirations. You can say your affirmations out loud, silently to yourself, or write them down.

Invest your affirmations with genuine feeling and back this up with a positive image of yourself. For example, you might see yourself surrounded by happy smiling friends, or imagine you are making a well-received presentation to colleagues, or excelling at your favourite sport.

Remember a time when you were particularly happy and felt good about yourself, and try to recapture those emotions. Tell yourself that you feel that way right now. By repeating these statements regularly they become imprinted on your subconscious and influence your conscious mind.

Social Support

When your symptoms are very severe, you might not feel like mixing with others. But if this situation carries on for a long time, you can lose contact with friends. You may then become socially isolated, and this can leave you depressed and make the symptoms worse.

Never underestimate the emotional support that partners, friends, family and work colleagues can provide. Being with people you like can lift your mood and counteract negative thoughts. Friends can offer a sympathetic ear when you feel low, and provide company when you feel isolated.

Friends and relatives may be reluctant to make the first move, especially if they sense that you are self-conscious about your symptoms. So always make the effort to keep in touch with them - at least by telephone. If you don't feel well enough to leave your home, invite them round to see you and, for example, watch a video or listen to music together - or just chat.

Be More Active

Choose a hobby, sport or pastime you can get absorbed in. It might be one you've been meaning to try but keep putting off. Or one you have neglected in recent years. Anything that occupies your thoughts in an enjoyable way will take your mind off your symptoms. And this, in turn, helps to alleviate them. Many pastimes put you in touch with people with a similar outlook and interests, and so increase your opportunities for making new friends.

Self-help Groups

There are IBS self-help groups you can join. It can be a great comfort to be with fellow sufferers who can empathize and offer comfort and support. For many people, attending a self-help group was the first opportunity they had had to get out of the house in a long time. Mixing with people who really understand can ease the sense of isolation and feelings of depression.

As well as listening to you, group members share their experiences with you, and offer hints and tips you can use. Self-help groups also keep members informed about the latest research into the causes of IBS, and about new medicines or other innovative treatments. Some self-help groups also provide one-to-one counselling for members (see Chapter Eleven).

Once IBS sufferers join a self-help group they experience a reduction in their symptoms and an improvement in general health. Studies show that the amount of medicine used reduces too, perhaps because they discover other ways of controlling their symptoms, or just feel much better.

However, studies have also shown that just talking about symptoms, although helpful, can become depressing and this is one reason why many members leave. To avoid this, many groups are run by trained counsellors who organize a structured programme. For example, each week the group may cover a different topic related to IBS.

If there is no self-help group in your area, you could ask the national support organization to help you set one up. Your doctor or local hospital can put you in contact with them, and with fellow sufferers.

Get Fit, Stay Fit

Regular moderate exercise provides numerous proven benefits - the most important (in the context of IBS) being that it can alleviate physical and mental symptoms. Many forms of exercise produce a powerful squeezing action on the bowel which - if you also consume plenty of fluid - helps break down solid, compacted stools and so relieves constipation.

Keeping fit also improves your physical health and mental well-being, giving you the energy, strength and suppleness to tackle work and domestic tasks with enthusiasm, and engender a more positive outlook on life.

Exercise stimulates release of the body's natural painkillers (endorphins) which suppress pain and lift mood. This counteracts negative mental states such as anxiety, depression and stress.

Exercise helps to counteract other symptoms and signs associated with stress, including muscular tension, insomnia, raised blood pressure and raised levels of glucose and fats in the blood. A keep-fit regime helps you to maintain a healthy diet and control your weight, so boosting self-image.

Several studies have shown that people notice a dramatic improvement in their mood and mental outlook within as little as three to five weeks of starting a regular exercise programme.

Boost Your Stamina

Keeping fit need not mean running marathons, or taking up gruelling weight-training programmes. In fact, quite the reverse. The healthiest forms of exercise are also the easiest. The key is to choose an activity that you can sustain at a moderate level for at least 30 minutes a session and are willing to repeat at least three or four times a week. If you have not exercised for a while, check with your doctor that regular exercise will be safe.

Brisk walking, steady jogging, cycling and swimming are all good forms of moderate stamina-building exercise. If you combine this with a general suppleness and toning regime, you should achieve a good level of fitness. Your local gym or fitness centre can suggest an exercise programme that is appropriate for you, or if you prefer to exercise on your own or with friends, you could buy an exercise video or keep-fit book.

There are other ways to increase your general fitness levels. You could take up a sport such as tennis or golf, or some other form of active pastime such as bird-watching, gardening or rambling/hiking. You could try to limit your car journeys. For example, for short journeys such as a visit to the local shop, church, club or pub, consider walking or cycling. Also try using the stairs rather than the lift, and walking up and down escalators rather than standing still on them.

Abdominal Exercises

There are specific abdominal exercises which you can practise each day to aid the passage of waste, ease constipation and reduce bowel spasms. Most keep-fit books and videos demonstrate appropriate exercises. The following have been adapted from yoga postures (see Chapter Twelve).

- Stand straight with your feet hip-width apart. Breathe in deeply, then bend forwards slightly and breathe out until you feel that you have emptied your lungs. Now contract your abdominal muscles and then relax them quickly. Repeat five times. Try to do this every day, steadily increasing the number of repetitions each day to a maximum of 15.

- Stand as before. Breathe in deeply, then bend forwards slightly and breathe out until you feel you have emptied your lungs. Contract your abdominal muscles and hold them in while you count to 10. Relax and breathe in. Repeat this four times.

- Lie down on your front and place your palms flat on the floor beneath your shoulders. Breathe in deeply, and breathe out until you feel you have emptied your lungs. Draw up your abdominal muscles. Pull your shoulders back and lift your head and shoulders off the ground. Now lift your abdomen off the floor. Hold while you count to five, then relax.

Pelvic Floor (Kegel) Exercises
Your pelvic floor is a collection of muscles, ligaments and other connective tissues that support the rectum, bladder, urethra, and - in women - vagina and uterus. By carrying out regular pelvic floor (or Kegel) exercises you can strengthen this structure and help to avoid urinary and faecal incontinence.

To find your pelvic floor, pretend you are trying to stop yourself breaking wind or have a full bladder but are trying to stop yourself urinating. As you do this you should feel a contraction around the bladder (and vagina) and a pulling sensation around the rectum - this indicates your pelvic floor.

Try to do the following exercises every day (you can do the exercises anywhere - even in public - as no one else will notice):

1. Contract and immediately relax your pelvic floor 10 times quickly.
2. Repeat, this time holding each contraction for a count of three and relaxing for a count of three. Over a period of weeks, you should be able to extend the contraction and relaxation phase to a count of ten.

Develop Good Bowel Habits
To encourage the bowel to function regularly and normally, it is not enough simply to strengthen your pelvic floor - you also need to develop good bowel habits. Most people have an urge to go to the toilet at least once each day, usually after they've eaten breakfast. You should never ignore this urge. Aim to visit the toilet as soon as you need to, and develop a daily routine.

Avoid Over-using Medications

You should avoid over-using medicines and recreational drugs as these can trigger IBS symptoms. For example, diarrhoea can be triggered by antacids or indigestion remedies that contain magnesium, by certain arthritis drugs and by laxatives. Constipation can be caused or made worse by antacids that contain aluminium or calcium, certain antidepressants and tranquillizers, iron tablets (in some people), painkillers and cough medicines that contain codeine (an opium derivative), and some types of drug given for bladder problems, abdominal pain and parkinsonism. Some hypertensives (medicines for high blood pressure) may cause diarrhoea or constipation. Avoid long-term use of laxatives, as you may become dependant on them.

If you think an over-the-counter remedy is making your symptoms worse, discontinue its use or ask your pharmacist to suggest an alternative. If you think a prescription medicine is to blame, talk to your doctor, who may prescribe a different form.

Caution
Never stop taking a prescription medicine without first consulting your doctor.

Recreational Drugs

The most widely used recreational drugs are cigarettes and alcohol, both known to aggravate IBS symptoms in some people. Alcohol and the nicotine in cigarettes can stimulate the chemoreceptors lining the bowel and trigger muscular spasms. Many illicit recreational drugs also disrupt the normal functioning of the bowel, leading to constipation and/or diarrhoea. These include: amphetamines such as 'speed', and barbiturates, cannabis, cocaine and opiate drugs such as opium, heroin and morphine.

Giving Up Smoking

If you have been planning to quit smoking, now is a good time to start. You will probably find your own method. But here are a few tips that have worked for other ex-smokers (including me):

● Set a date for giving up when you don't expect to be under extra stress. For example, don't try to quit when you are facing exams, changing jobs or moving house.

● Tell friends, relatives and colleagues when you plan to give up. This will strengthen your resolve and (hopefully) they will support you.

● During the preceding week, reduce the number of cigarettes you smoke each day, and smoke the last one the night before you plan to quit.

- For the first few weeks avoid alcohol, tea and coffee - which increase your craving. Drink fruit or vegetable juices and herbal drinks instead.
- Eat plenty of fresh fruit and vegetables, and buy or prepare healthy snacks such as chopped raw vegetables, fruit pieces, pretzels or low-fat bread sticks.
- Change your routine to avoid pubs, clubs and other places that you normally associate with smoking.
- Spend more time at social venues where smoking is not allowed, such as cinemas and theatres.
- Devote the early evening to a physical activity such as a session in the gym, playing sport, swimming or going for a long walk or cycle ride. This will take your mind off smoking and boost your endorphin levels, which will counteract your cravings. It will also help you to sleep (but don't exercise too late or it can keep you awake - see Chapter Eight).
- Keep busy to take your mind off smoking - this might be a good time to decorate the spare bedroom, tidy the garage or clear out the loft.

If you can't quit, try to limit your smoking as much as possible and consider using nicotine patches instead of cigarettes on occasion (not nicotine gum, which you may find has the same effect on your bowel as smoking).

Cutting Down on Alcohol
You could try avoiding all forms of alcohol for a while to see what effect this has on your symptoms. Otherwise, try to moderate your intake to no more than two glasses of beer, wine or spirits a day, and have two or three alcohol-free days each week.

A good way to reduce your drinking is to find low-alcohol or non-alcoholic substitutes. If you don't want to give up alcohol completely, try different kinds to see if that makes a difference. (White wine is a common trigger for IBS symptoms, so if this is your tipple you might switch to something else.)

- In restaurants, drink water or fruit juice instead of wine with your meals.
- At parties, ask the host to make a non-alcoholic punch or cocktails from fruit and vegetable juices - and encourage others to have some.
- In clubs and pubs, have a shandy or ask for low-alcohol beer.
- Dilute your drinks. For example, drink spritzers (wine and soda) instead of drinking wine neat, and add a mixer such as tonic or lemonade to spirits.

Case Study: Mick

Mick, 39, is a heating contractor. He had suffered IBS symptoms for several years before his wife persuaded him to see his doctor: 'I think part of my trouble is that I'm always in a hurry. I know I should sit down and take more time over my meals but I'm self-employed and often I only have time to grab a pie or a sandwich. My wife says that even when I sit down to a meal she's cooked I just wolf it down without tasting it. My doctor said that if I really worked on my diet and took more time over my meals it would help. My wife packs me my lunch now, usually a wholemeal bread sandwich, and always some fruit, or some pieces of raw vegetable. And I have a fruit drink with it. I try not to rush now. I usually take a break for at least half an hour to digest my meals. I think it's helping.'

Chapter Six

Foods to Avoid

Many IBS sufferers find that certain foods and drinks regularly trigger symptoms. For example, spicy, rich or fatty foods, coffee, tea, fizzy drinks (including gassy beers such as lager) and even chewing gum can cause symptoms such as cramping pain, excess wind and an urgent need to go to the toilet. You can help to manage your symptoms by identifying problem foods and avoiding (or cutting down on) them, and finding suitable alternatives.

Identifying Problem Foods

If you don't want to keep an IBS diary (see Chapter Five), you can simply note down which foods you eat and when, or keep to a strict weekly menu. Then, if symptoms are worse on certain days, you will have narrowed down the list of 'suspects'. Another way is with an elimination diet. In essence, this involves keeping to foods that rarely cause symptoms. After 2-3 weeks, if your symptoms have improved, you can introduce suspect foods one at a time, to see if symptoms recur.

Once an elimination diet helps you to discover which foods you can tolerate and which you must avoid, you can reintroduce some of the items previously on your 'banned' list. The following foods are thought unlikely to cause symptoms, and so can form the basis of your elimination diet:

- meat and fish: chicken and turkey (excluding the skin, which contains the fat); white fish
- starchy foods: buckwheat, millet, plain rice (including rice cakes and rice flour), sago and tapioca
- vegetables: but excluding potatoes, onions, sweetcorn and pulses
- fruits: except citrus fruits and grapefruit (and their juices)
- drinks: herbal teas, most fruit juices (but not citrus) and mineral water.

Check with Your Doctor

Before eliminating problem foods you should discuss your plans with your doctor, in case there is any medical reason why an exclusion diet may not be advisable in your case. If your doctor has no objections, he or she may recommend a dietitian or nutritionist who can suggest a diet that ensures you avoid problematic foods and yet still obtain the nourishment you need.

Limiting Problem Foods

In some cases it may be only one or two food items that trigger symptoms. If so, it should be easy to avoid them. To check that they were causing a problem, simply cut them out of your diet for a few weeks, then reintroduce them. If your symptoms recur, you will know those foods were responsible.

You may not need to avoid all problem foods. You might find that simply by reducing the amount of certain foods you eat you can still have a varied and enjoyable diet while keeping your symptoms under control.

For example, fatty meats can trigger or exacerbate IBS symptoms in some people. But meat itself is a good source of protein, vitamins and minerals. You can reduce your fat intake simply by choosing less fatty types or leaner cuts, removing excess fat and using cooking methods such as boiling, grilling, stir-frying and steaming that reduce the fat content and add little or no extra fat or oil to the meal.

Allergies and Sensitivities

Some people develop IBS-like symptoms because of an allergy or sensitivity to certain foodstuffs. A food allergy is a severe, inappropriate reaction by the body's immune system towards a particular foodstuff. Some of the most common allergy triggers (allergens) are nuts, especially peanuts, shellfish and strawberries.

Food sensitivities, on the other hand, are most often caused by a deficiency of an important enzyme or an inability to absorb a particular component in a food. Perhaps the best-known examples of food sensitivities are coeliac disease and lactose intolerance.

Coeliac disease is a hypersensitivity reaction to gluten, a protein found in cereals such as wheat, oats, rye and barley. As a result, the lining of the gut becomes inflamed and damaged and is less efficient at absorbing all nutrients, not just those in cereals. Sufferers have to avoid all foods that contain gluten (including biscuits and cakes made with gluten wheat).

Lactose is a disaccharide sugar found in milk. Lactose intolerance is caused by a deficiency of the enzyme lactase in the body, which is needed to digest this sugar. Lactase is produced in large quantities in infants and small children, but levels tend to decline in adults. World-wide, around 75 per cent of the adult population cannot digest lactose at all. If lactose is not digested in the small bowel, the sugar passes through to the large bowel where intestinal bacteria break it down, producing large amounts of carbon dioxide and hydrogen.

Boycotting Bread
Some nutritionists say an allergy or intolerance to wheat and milk is the underlying cause of a number of common medical disorders, including IBS. The theory is controversial. There is little evidence to show that IBS is caused by an allergic reaction or enzyme deficiency. Nevertheless, many IBS sufferers find their symptoms improve if they avoid wheat and milk. It may be that, in IBS sufferers, chemoreceptors in the bowel react more violently to gluten, or lactose, or some other substance.

Life without Wheat
Gluten is not only found in bread made with wheat, but in any wheat-based product, including batter, biscuits, cake, pastries, packet soups and sausages. You'll need to check the list of ingredients on any processed food you buy to see whether it contains wheat flour in some form. Health shops stock gluten-free bread, flour and pasta. And there are many other types of wholegrains, and other foods, you can try instead (see Chapter Seven).

Dodging Dairy
Although dairy products are often linked with IBS symptoms, this may be as much because of their generally high fat content as for the lactose they contain. The best-known dairy foods are milk, butter, cream and cheese. But many processed foods such as puddings, ready meals, sauces, biscuits and other snacks can contain 'hidden' lactose and other milk-derived ingredients. These may be listed as milk solids, skimmed milk powder, whey solids and whey. Bear in mind that all forms of milk contain lactose, whether from a cow, a goat or a sheep. The main differences between, say, cow's and goat's milk is the amount of fat and types of protein they contain.

Dairy foods are a major source of calcium, needed for healthy teeth, bones and nerves, as well as protein, vitamin B2 and zinc. So if you decide to abstain from all dairy products, to see if your symptoms improve, it is a good idea to find healthy replacements. For example, soya milk and rice milk are nutritious alternatives to cow's milk (see Chapter Seven).

Sweeteners
Some artificial sweeteners should be avoided if you have diarrhoea, but may be useful if you have constipation. Sorbitol and xylitol, for example, cannot be digested by the body's own digestive enzymes. Bacteria feed on these substances and produce acids which irritate the lining of the bowel,

causing the release of copious amounts of water and leading to looser, more frequent stools. Sorbitol is found in some sweets, sugar-free chewing gum, jams and other preserves, and special foods made for people with diabetes.

Wind-generators

Some foods generate a great deal of gas, exacerbating the problem of abdominal distension and flatulence. The best-known 'wind-generators' are beans and other pulses (such as peas, lentils and chickpeas) which can cause bloating and excess gas. Other problem foods include:

- cruciferous vegetables (members of the cabbage family, including broccoli, Brussels sprouts and cauliflower)
- asafoetida, a herb of the fennel family (used in Indian meals)
- members of the onion family, including garlic and leeks
- root vegetables such as swedes and turnips
- seeds, including poppy and sunflower.

Cruciferous vegetables are rich in important nutrients, however. As well as fibre, they contain vitamins C and E and folate, to guard against heart disease, and minerals such as calcium, iron and potassium, for healthy bones, teeth and nerves. They also contain sulphur compounds, or glucosinolates, which become anti-cancer chemicals inside the body.

Rather than give up such foods completely, it may be sufficient just to lower your intake until your flatulence is manageable. (Remember, it is not possible to eliminate all gas, even in non-IBS sufferers.) You only need an average intake of 30 g (1 oz) of cruciferous vegetables per day to get the optimum amount of nutrients you need.

Caffeine

This mildly addictive sedative drug is found in a surprising number of products, not only tea and coffee but also some types of chocolate, carbonated drinks and many types of painkiller. It can cause diarrhoea, spasms and an urgent desire to go. Because it interferes with the brain's anti-pain system, it can also intensify pain. Decaffeinated coffee can also cause symptoms in some people.

Other Problem Foods and Drinks

Other foods known to aggravate IBS symptoms in some people include:
- alcohol (especially white wine)
- carbonated (fizzy) drinks
- chocolate

- citrus fruits (such as oranges, lemons, satsumas, mandarins, clementines)
- eggs (and products - such as cakes - made with them)
- maize (including corn-on-the cob)
- potatoes
- red and green peppers (containing the chemical capsaicin, which can cause your bowel to go into spasm)
- rich or fatty foods (all fried food, burgers, sausages and other fatty meats, cream cakes and rich sauces)
- table sugar (or sucrose, often added to sweet *and* savoury processed foods; excess sucrose is acted on by bacteria in the bowel, causing gas and triggering other symptoms).

Planning a Healthy Diet

You must take care not to exclude too many important foods. Any radical change in diet must be carefully planned to ensure that it provides all the nutrients you need. A healthy diet should include:
- Starchy carbohydrates, for example from bread, flour, rice, pasta, potatoes and maize. This type of food should make up the bulk of your diet.
- Proteins, for example from meat, fish and pulses such as lentils, peas, beans and nuts. If you are vegetarian you should eat as wide a range of protein-rich plant foods as possible. This will ensure that you get all the essential amino acids (the 'building blocks' from which proteins are made) that your body needs.
- Fats and oils, for example from dairy foods, margarine, nuts and seeds (and oils made from them), meat and oily fish (such as herring, mackerel, tuna and salmon). These should be eaten sparingly. By eating a range of fats and oils (in small amounts) you will get all the kinds (known as Essential Fatty Acids) needed for good health.
- Fruit and vegetables. Eat plenty of different kinds to get the vitamins and minerals you need.

Detox Diets
Many nutritionists say that disorders like IBS may be caused, in part, by increased gut 'permeability', leading to raised levels of toxins in the body. In effect, the gut - including the bowel - becomes more porous and so allows through more toxins, such as pesticides and other pollutants, than the liver can render safe.

This theory is highly controversial, as is the suggested solution - 'detox' (short for detoxification). Detox usually takes the form of a strict diet, usually involving fruit and vegetable juices and a limited range of relatively bland foods (along with the avoidance of 'toxic' substances such as caffeine, cigarettes and alcohol). A detox diet may also include a fast, lasting one or more days.

Fasting is not recommended if you are ill, malnourished, finding it difficult to eat or have a serious medical condition, and any change in diet should be supervised by a registered dietitian or doctor. This applies especially to people with diabetes, who must maintain a strict dietary regime in order to regulate their blood sugar levels.

The majority of irritable bowel sufferers, however, are well nourished and in generally good health - apart from their symptoms. So a detox diet may be beneficial. Psychologically, a detox diet can be useful in giving you a sense of 'empowerment' by enabling you to do something positive to improve your condition. It can also make it easier to cut down or avoid substances such as caffeine, alcohol, cigarettes and fatty or spicy foods which trigger symptoms. The fresh fruits and vegetables you eat can only be a good thing. And a detox diet may help you make a permanent switch to a healthier and better-balanced diet.

A Detox Regime

The following five-day detox regime includes a one-day fast (on day 3). A healthy, well-nourished person can easily fast for a day (provided he or she drinks plenty of fluids) without serious ill-effects. However, one side-effect of fasting may be a temporary drop in energy, leading to fatigue or lethargy.

You may also suffer mild headaches as a result of going without tea, coffee and fizzy drinks. (Headache is a common symptom of caffeine withdrawal.) If you choose to follow this diet, choose a time, such as a holiday, when you can take it easy for a while.

The following regime may include foods you've not tried before (see Chapter Seven). If you like them, you could make them a regular part of your diet. If you know that any of these foods can trigger symptoms (or have other adverse effects), simply replace them with foods you can tolerate.

Day 1   Plan meals using any of the following: buckwheat, brown rice, fish, lentils, millet, quinoa, soya products (including tofu, soya flour and soya milk), olive oil, plain unsweetened live yoghurt and as many fresh fruits and vegetables as you like. Drink only water, herbal teas, soya milk and fresh fruit or vegetable juices (but not citrus juices). Avoid convenience foods, fried foods, dairy products (except live yoghurt), eggs, meat, wheat products (such as bread and pasta), table salt, sugar, chocolate, tea, coffee, alcohol and, of course, cigarettes.

Day 2   Eat only fruits, vegetables and plain, unsweetened live yoghurt. Drink plenty of fluids such as water, herbal teas and fruit or vegetable juices.

Day 3   Avoid solid food but be sure to drink plenty of fluids (at least 4 litres/7 pints) such as water, herbal teas and fresh fruit or vegetable juices.

Day 4   As for Day 2.

Day 5   As for Day 1.

You can now return to your normal diet if you wish, but to consolidate the beneficial effects of the detox regime, include as many of the foods listed on the first day (especially fresh fruit and vegetables, and juices made from them) and limit your intake of items on the 'avoid' list.

It is now time to look at the healthy, delicious and nutritious foods you could try to help manage your IBS symptoms. This is the subject of Chapter Seven.

Case Study: Sonia
Sonia found that medication helped control her symptoms but caused other problems: 'The medication [an antispasmodic] stops me being constipated. The problem is that now I go to the loo far more regularly - several times a day - and not always at the most convenient times. Also, every time I eat something the food passes through ever so quickly. I have to take my medication 30 minutes before I have a meal. But 30 minutes after I have eaten I get very bad cramping pains and diarrhoea and then I worry that I won't be able to get to the toilet. There are times when I can't go out and I have to be careful about journey times. But I've pretty much sorted out what foods cause it - wheat, pasta, chips, spicy food, chocolate and anything rich - especially couscous. The trouble is, the foods I like seem to cause most problems. I can't try anything new in a restaurant in case it triggers an attack. I went out for dinner with my parents and I chose a starter I'd never tried before. Unfortunately, I got such terrible pains that we had to go home.'

Chapter Seven

What Foods Should You Eat?

The aim of any change to your diet should be to introduce any new foods slowly, to give your body time to adjust. This applies particularly to adding more fibre to your diet, the single most important change you can make to help alleviate your symptoms.

If you're used to low-fibre meals, it can be difficult to switch to fibre-rich foods. For one thing, it means cutting down on some favourite foods and eating others you might not like so much. The extra fibre in your diet may even make your symptoms worse, for a while.

You need to find the right level of fibre for you - enough to alleviate symptoms, but not so much that it causes other problems. It is well worth persevering with a high-fibre diet, however. Any problems should ease off after a few weeks. Most people see an improvement within four weeks.

Defining Fibre

'Fibre' is the term used to describe the parts of plant foods that cannot be broken down by human digestive enzymes. Fibre is known by other names too, such as 'roughage' and 'non-starch polysaccharide' (or NSP). Some of these terms are misleading: 'fibre' does not always look 'fibrous', and 'roughage' is not usually 'rough' (in the sense of being abrasive) but often smooth. However, 'fibre' is the term most people are familiar with.

There are three main types of fibre:
1. cellulose, found mainly in unprocessed cereals
2. pectins, found in most fruit and vegetables
3. mucilage, found in pulses (such as peas, chickpeas, beans and lentils) and some cereals.

Cellulose does not dissolve in water and so is also called 'insoluble fibre'. By speeding the passage of faeces through the bowel, insoluble fibre limits the amount of time that cancer-causing chemicals (carcinogens) in the waste stay in contact with the bowel lining. This may be one reason why the peoples of African countries, where high-fibre diets are the norm, have low rates of bowel cancer compared with the West.

Pectins and mucilage do dissolve in water, and so are known as 'soluble fibre' (as they turn into gels they are also known as 'gel-forming fibres'). Mucilage is beneficial in IBS because it lubricates and soothes the bowel lining.

All soluble fibre binds with cholesterol in the bile salts which the liver secretes into the gut, and prevents its reabsorption into the bloodstream. This reduces blood levels of 'bad' cholesterol (low-density lipoproteins, or LDLs) and cuts the risk of heart disease and strokes. This is useful, as cholesterol levels are often raised in people who suffer stress - a common problem in IBS.

Soluble fibre also slows down the rate at which carbohydrate is digested and absorbed into the bloodstream. This helps regulate blood sugar levels and so protects against type II, non-insulin dependent (or mature-onset) diabetes mellitus (a common form of diabetes, affecting mainly older people).

The most important characteristic of fibre is that it is 'hydrophilic' - it absorbs water and swells - by up to 15 times - providing the bulk needed to propel waste through the bowel. Also, by absorbing such copious amounts of water, fibre keeps waste soft and malleable and stops hard, compacted stools forming.

As fibre slowly expands it keeps the bowel walls slightly distended and helps to control the spasms that trigger symptoms such as pain, bloating and diarrhoea.

Good Sources of Fibre

The modern diet is made up of a lot of convenience and snack foods that have lost much of their fibre during processing. Nutritionists say that a healthy diet should contain a daily intake of around 18 g (just over half an ounce) of fibre. However, most people in the West eat only around 12 g. The best way to get the fibre you need is to eat more unprocessed plant foods, such as fruit, vegetables, pulses and wholegrains:

The Amount of Fibre (per 100 g) in Many Common Foods

Food	Grams of fibre (per 100 g)
Cereals	
brown rice	1
Corn Flakes	1
wholemeal bread	6
wholemeal flour	9
bran breakfast cereal	15

Food	Grams of fibre (per 100 g)

Cereals cont.

buckwheat	16
wheat bran	36

Vegetables

celery	1
plum tomatoes (tinned)	1
lettuce	1
sweetcorn	1.5
leeks	2
spinach	2
spring greens	2
carrots	3
jacket potato	3
avocado	3.5
parsnips	4.5

Fresh fruit

apples	2
pears	2
raspberries	3
strawberries	3
blackberries	3
blueberries	3

Dried fruit

raisins	1.2
sultanas	1.2
apricots (semi-dried)	6
prunes (semi-dried)	6
figs (dried)	8

Pulses

baked beans	5
peas	5
haricot beans (boiled)	6
broad beans	7
kidney beans	7
red lentils	7

Food	Grams of fibre (per 100 g)

Nuts

walnuts	3.5
brazil nuts	4
peanuts	4-6
almonds	7
hazelnuts	7
coconut (desiccated)	14

Increasing Your Fibre Intake

To include more fibre in your diet, why not try the following?:

- Eat porridge, a bran or wholegrain cereal, or toast made with whole-grain bread for breakfast.
- Snack on raw vegetables such as asparagus, sliced carrot, pieces of broccoli and cauliflower (to make them more palatable, eat with a fat-free dip).
- Eat plain fruit as a snack or for pudding - and try different types and mixtures of fruit.
- Eat dried fruit as a tasty snack or sprinkled over breakfast cereal.
- Add cooked beans, lentils, peas and grated or sliced vegetables to casseroles, stews, salads, sauces and soups.

Fibre Supplements

As well as eating high-fibre foods, you can add extra fibre to meals in the form of bran, linseed and psyllium.

Caution
Drink plenty of fluids with your meals and throughout the day when taking these supplements.

Bran

Bran is the husk from wheat and oat grains that is usually discarded when cereals are processed to make white flour. Bran has the highest fibre content of any food substance. It can be added to bread and breakfast cereals, sprinkled over meals, stirred into stews and casseroles, or used medicinally (see ChapterTen).Wheat bran and oat bran produce less gas than other types of fibre. But in people who are wheat-sensitive or wheat-intolerant, these are probably best avoided. Alternatives are rice bran and soya bran, available from health food stores.

Linseed (or Flaxseed, *Linum usitatissimum*)
This nutritious seed contains soluble fibre, to add bulk, and insoluble fibre, to soothe the lining of the bowel. The newer, tastier golden linseed is particularly popular. Linseed can be sprinkled over foods after cooking or ground up and added to cereals. You can also mix 1 teaspoon of ground seeds with around 250 ml (half a pint) of water or fruit juice and drink up to three times a day. Linseed is a good source of omega-3 essential fatty acids, vitamin E and iron. It is especially rich in vitamin E, but can go rancid if kept for too long. So buy only a few days' supply at a time and store in a fridge or freezer until needed.

Psyllium
Psyllium is a gel-forming soluble fibre made from the seed husks of the psyllium plant (*Plantago ovata*). It is used in many bulk laxatives and added to some breakfast cereals. It is available from health food stores. You can mix up to 1 tablespoon of psyllium husks or powder into 250 ml (approximately half a pint) of water and drink once a day about half an hour after a meal. Drink the mixture immediately, before it starts to thicken. As psyllium is high in soluble fibre it can also reduce blood cholesterol levels.

Fibre Problems

Some people feel better as soon as they start eating high-fibre foods. But for others, getting the balance right is tricky. Don't despair if changing your diet doesn't bring immediate benefits. You may even find that your symptoms (such as bloating, abdominal distension, flatulence and diarrhoea) get worse during the first few weeks. In part this may be due to the fact that eating more fibre affects the balance of bacteria in the gut.

To prevent this, increase your fibre intake slowly. This allows time for bacteria in the bowel to adjust. If your symptoms get worse, reduce the amount of fibre or try other kinds. Include just enough fibre in your diet to produce stools that are soft, painless and easily passed.

Instead of completely switching to brown rice, wholemeal pasta or wholegrain flour, you could add a little of the high-fibre types to the low-fibre kinds you are used to. For example, mix brown rice with white rice in a ratio of 1:3. As your bowel gets used to it, increase the ratio to 2:2 and then 3:1 until you can phase out the white rice. If this triggers symptoms, simply reduce the amount of brown rice. You can use the same approach with wholemeal pasta.

If you make your own bread, you can include as much wholegrain flour as you want (a breadmaker is ideal for this). For store-bought bread, start with one slice of wholegrain bread per every (say) three slices of white bread you have, and steadily increase the ratio of wholegrain.

Avoid Excess Fibre

Don't go to the other extreme and overdo your fibre intake drastically, as this causes problems too, such as intestinal blockage - especially if you don't drink enough water. Fibre also binds with some nutrients and prevents absorption. However, provided you keep to a well-balanced diet that includes plenty of fruits and vegetables, this should not be a problem.

All large stores and health food shops stock an impressive range of wholegrain and other fibre-, vitamin- and mineral-rich foods which you may have been tempted to try in the past. We'll now look at these foods in detail.

Healthy Foods to Eat

Most IBS sufferers feel better when they change to a healthier diet. Probably the most important steps you can take, apart from eating natural, unprocessed foods such as fruits, vegetables and wholegrains, is to drink more water and other fluids. Dried fruit and live yoghurt can also make an important contribution to your diet.

Water of Life

Water is important for everyone, but especially so for IBS sufferers. People with C-IBS need to drink lots of water to soften the stool and facilitate its passage through the bowel. Those with D-IBS need to stay well hydrated to replace the large amount of fluid they lose every time they pass loose, watery stools.

It is especially important to drink plenty of fluids with meals whenever you increase the amount of fibre in your diet, or use laxatives (see Chapter Ten). Otherwise, high-fibre foods or laxatives will make your constipation worse and your bowel can even become dangerously impacted.

You should also have regular drinks throughout the day. Don't wait until you feel thirsty to have a drink. Thirst is not an accurate indicator of your body's requirements. By the time your brain 'tells' you that you need a fluid 'top-up', you are probably already dehydrated.

A better guide to your fluid levels is the colour of your urine, which should be pale yellow - or virtually clear. Dark, amber-coloured urine is caused by a build-up of urea, a waste product derived from the breakdown of proteins. Urea is produced by the body at a steady rate, so a build-up shows you're not urinating enough.

All adults should aim to drink at least 2 litres (3 $^1/_2$ pints) of fluids a day, but you may need even more than this - especially when:

- you are pregnant or breastfeeding
- the weather is hot or humid
- you are exercising
- you have a digestive disorder
- you have diarrhoea
- you have been vomiting.

What to Drink

Pure water is the best drink of all. Whether you choose bottled or tap water, or boiled water that has been allowed to cool, is up to you. You can improve the taste of plain water by flavouring it with lemon or lime juice, freshly picked mint leaves or ginger.

Other good ways to increase your fluid intake include drinking herbal teas and fruit or vegetable juices. (To avoid tooth decay, dilute fruit juices to make them less acidic.) Many people find that peppermint herbal tea can alleviate IBS symptoms such as abdominal pain. Cut down on caffeinated drinks and alcohol - they not only aggravate IBS symptoms but also cause you to urinate more and so make you dehydrated.

Natural is Best

Food processing - especially milling and refining - not only removes fibre, it also strips out nutrients that guard against disease. By eating more natural foods you not only get more fibre but also obtain the vitamins and minerals that help prevent, for example, anaemia, high blood pressure, heart disease, diabetes and cancer.

Natural foods are rich in:

- antioxidants, such as beta carotene and vitamins C and E, which protect against heart disease and cancer
- B vitamins, for healthy nerves and muscles and speedy recovery from illness and injury
- calcium for strong teeth and bones
- folate (folic acid), for a healthy heart and blood vessels (also vital for women of child-bearing age to prevent spina bifida in the unborn baby)
- iron, an important component of red blood cells (people who are lacking in this mineral suffer iron-deficiency anaemia)
- magnesium, for strong bones and healthy cell function

- omega-3 essential fatty acids, which help reduce blood levels of LDL
- phytoestrogens, plant hormones that protect against some cancers
- potassium, which helps to regulate high blood pressure
- zinc, for a healthy immune system and rapid wound healing.

Wholegrains for Health

Many types of wholegrains are available from grocery stores and health shops. As well as unrefined wheat and oats (if you can tolerate them), you could try rye, buckwheat, millet, pot barley and quinoa. Pot barley, unlike pearl barley, retains its husk and has five times as much fibre as wheat.

Nutritionists say that starchy foods like wholegrains (and also noodles, brown rice, pasta and potatoes) should make up about half of the daily calorie intake. They are not only high in fibre, but also highly nutritious.

Wheat Alternatives

If wheat-based bread triggers symptoms, try rye bread, or bread made with rice flour. If you are avoiding all grains containing gluten, you could try brown rice, buckwheat, corn, millet (sorghum), quinoa and wild rice. In some people, an adverse reaction to bread is not caused by wheat itself, but by the additives, preservatives and bleaching agents it contains. You can buy flour that is free from additives (but goes stale quickly!).

Brown Rice

This is an excellent energy food and, as it contains the husk that is lost during the refining of white rice, a good source of fibre and nutrients such as thiamin (vitamin B1). The Western diet is low in thiamin, an important vitamin for healthy nerves, and white rice contains hardly any at all. Rice can be ground into flour, and made into rice bread and rice cakes, or turned into rice milk - a good alternative to cow's milk. Brown basmati rice is a fragrant type of rice, used in Asian dishes, and the easiest rice to cook.

Buckwheat

Despite the name, buckwheat is not related to wheat. It's not even a cereal. It comes from the seed of the *Fagopyrum* genus and is related to rhubarb. It is an important food for vegetarians because it contains lysine, an essential amino acid not found in most plant foods. Buckwheat is also a source of the antioxidants selenium and vitamin A and is rich in rutin, which helps maintain a healthy heart and blood vessels. Buckwheat grains can be cooked like rice, or turned into flour and used to make griddle-baked flat bread (galettes), crepes and noodles.

Corn

This versatile grain is also known as corn on the cob, grits, maize, polenta, popcorn and sweetcorn. It is turned into myriad forms including corn flour, corn oil and corn syrup. In its unrefined form, ground cornmeal, it retains all of its nutrients. It can be made into quick breads, puddings and cakes, or served up as an accompaniment to meat and fish dishes.

Millet

This is a staple of Asia, North Africa and southern Europe. As well as being high in fibre, it contains essential amino acids, vitamins and minerals. It can be added to soups, stews and casseroles.

Quinoa

Strictly speaking, quinoa is not a grain but the fruit of a South American herb. It is ideal for vegetarians because it contains all the amino acids needed for good health, as well as minerals including potassium and iron, and B vitamins. It can be served as an accompaniment to other dishes.

Wild Rice

Despite the name, this is actually the seed of a wild aquatic grass grown in North America. It is rich in amino acids and B vitamins and can be cooked like rice and served up as an accompaniment to many dishes, or mixed with standard brown rice.

Pulses for Protein

All pulses, including beans, peas and lentils, are a good source of soluble and insoluble fibre, as well as being high in protein and important minerals. Pulses come well down the typical Western diet, and yet are highly nutritious, providing around 7 g of fibre per 100 g.

As well as being important for healthy bowel function, the fibre in pulses helps stabilize blood sugar levels, prevent heart disease and lower LDL ('bad') cholesterol levels in the blood. Pulses are a rich source of protein and so provide a useful non-fat alternative to meat in the diet. In addition, most pulses are high in folate, calcium, potassium, iron and zinc.

Pulses most widely available include aduki beans, black-eyed beans, butter beans, chickpeas, mung beans, pinto beans, red kidney beans, and red and brown lentils. Red lentils can be bought whole or split. The split kind, which don't need soaking, are the most widely available in the West.

Some beans, such as red kidney beans and broad beans, need to be well cooked to neutralize certain harmful chemicals. Follow the cooking instructions on the packet, or buy tinned (and hence ready-cooked) kinds.

Some people find pulses rather indigestible, however, and they can cause excess gas and bloating. If you find this a problem you should reduce your intake, or perhaps avoid them altogether.

A way to make pulses less problematic is to allow them to germinate and produce sprouts. This converts some of their starch into more easily digestible sugar. To germinate lentils, soak them overnight in tepid water. Drain and replace with fresh tepid water and leave for a further four hours. Drain again and place the lentils between layers of damp kitchen paper and leave in a dark place, making sure they stay damp. After 36 hours, small sprouts will develop. The lentils are now ready to eat. To cook, stir fry in a little vegetable oil and serve piping hot as an accompaniment to rice dishes.

Soya - The Versatile Bean

Soya is actually a pulse, but it is such a useful food it deserves a separate mention. The Chinese call soya 'meat without bones' because of the bean's high protein content. It is also packed with soluble and insoluble fibre and is a source of calcium, folate, iron, manganese, potassium, vitamin E and zinc. It offers a good alternative to animal products if you're trying to cut down on meat. In studies, people who replaced some of the meat in meals with soya bean products had much reduced levels of LDL cholesterol and so were at far lower risk of heart disease.

The low rate of breast cancer in Japan is attributed, in part, to the fact that the Japanese diet is high in soya and low in dairy produce. It is thought that a high level of oestrogen (the female sex hormone) is a risk factor in breast cancer. Soya is a good source of phytoestrogens - a weak plant form of oestrogen that does not cause breast cancer but does make the body reduce the human oestrogen in the blood to safer levels.

Soya is extremely versatile. As a flour it can be formed and flavoured for use as a meat substitute. For people who find that dairy products aggravate their symptoms, soya milk is a good alternative in beverages, cooking or as a refreshing drink on its own. Unlike animal milk, soya milk does not contain the natural sugar lactose and so can seem rather bland. Some brands of soya milk are sweetened with apple juice to make them more palatable.

Soya can be turned into tofu, which, when made with the setting agent calcium chloride, is a good non-dairy source of calcium. Tofu can be used in Western recipes as a meat or cheese substitute, as well as in patés, sauces and soups. It can be boiled, sautéed, steamed and stir-fried. Soya is also fermented as miso, a soya bean paste, and tempeh, a solid product with a nutty taste that can be sliced and fried, or chopped up and added to casseroles and other dishes.

Fresh Fruit and Vegetables

All fresh fruit and vegetables are good sources of fibre, especially soluble kinds. High levels of pectins are found in apples, blackberries, blackcurrants, pears and quinces. Vegetables are most nutritious when eaten raw or only lightly cooked. Eating the skins of potatoes (for example as jacket potato), and some fruit and vegetables every day, increases your intake of insoluble fibre.

Dried Fruit
Dried fruits contain soluble and insoluble fibre and are useful - and delicious - additions to any diet. They can be incorporated into breakfast cereals and puddings, or eaten as a low-fat snack between meals. All dried fruit, but especially apricots, dates, figs and prunes, help alleviate constipation when consumed with fluid to help them swell.

Homemade Laxative
You can make an effective laxative using 1 cup of apple sauce, 1 cup of prune juice and 1 cup of wheat bran. Mix together well and store in the fridge. Take 2 tablespoons each evening and then drink a large glass of water. This should help you to have a regular bowel movement. After the first week, if there is little improvement, increase to up to 4 tablespoons.

Important
Drink plenty of fluid when taking this, or any, laxative.

Bacterial Boost

There is another advantage in eating fibre-rich foods. Insoluble fibre encourages the growth of beneficial bacteria in the bowel, which is helpful in keeping harmful (or pathogenic) micro-organisms at bay. You can also boost levels of 'friendly gut flora' by including live yoghurt in your diet.

Yoghurt - Gut Guardian

Yoghurt is a good source of calcium and other vital nutrients, but its main asset is that it contains bacteria that can improve the health of the bowel. These include *Bifidobacterium longum*, *Lactobacillus acidophilus* and *Streptococcus*. Many brands of yoghurt have been pasteurized (heat-treated) to kill off the bacteria, so check the label says 'live' bacteria before buying.

Yoghurt bacteria can keep in check pathogens such as *Escherichia coli*,

Campylobacteria and the yeast fungus *Candida albicans*. Candida, which also causes the throat and vaginal infection candidiasis or 'thrush', is found in the bowel of around 50 per cent of the population in the West.

Recent research suggests that symbiotic (helpful) micro-organisms act by:

- preventing pathogens from attaching themselves to the bowel lining
- producing chemicals that inhibit both the pathogens and the toxins that pathogens secrete
- stimulating antibodies that attack the pathogens
- allowing time for the bowel's own beneficial flora to build up numbers.

The bowel's 'floral' balance is easily disrupted. Not only do antibiotics kill off friendly bacteria, but corticosteroid drugs (used to treat inflammatory conditions) can suppress the immune system. This allows pathogens in the gut to multiply, irritating the bowel lining and causing IBS symptoms. Eating live yoghurt on a regular basis helps restore optimum levels of the body's own useful microbes, and prevents pathogens gaining a foothold.

Although dairy products pose problems for some people, live yoghurt is usually well tolerated. This may be because the micro-organisms in yoghurt supply the enzyme lactase, needed to digest lactose.

If you can't tolerate live yoghurt, you can obtain 'probiotic' supplements of gut bacteria such as *Bifidobacteria longum*, *Enterococcus faecium*, *Lactobacillus acidophilus*, *L. bulgaricus*, *L. reutteri* and *L. rhamnosus GG*. These are available at health food stores. A typical intake is $1/2$-1 tsp of one or more types in a glass of mineral water, taken two or three times a day. The probiotic yeast *Saccharomyces boulardii* can also be beneficial.

In one study, significantly more IBS patients showed an improvement in symptoms after taking supplements of Lactobacilli, when compared with a control group who were given medication only. (Bifidobacterium supplements have also been used to treat ulcerative colitis, a disorder which - unlike IBS - causes inflammation of the bowel wall. It was found that ulcerative colitis patients tend to lack this bacterium in their gut.)

Tasty Healthy Recipes

The following recipe ideas contain lots of foods that are high in fibre and plant proteins, and have many other nutrients to ensure a well-balanced meal. These recipes include ingredients which are usually well-tolerated by IBS sufferers. However, if any of these foods trigger your symptoms, simply replace them with suitable alternatives. The metric and imperial measures shown are not exact conversions, so follow one or the other, but not both.

Fruity Muesli

The dried fruits in this recipe can be varied according to taste or availability - or mixed together - but try to keep the ratio of grains to fruit the same. Dry muesli will keep fresh for several weeks if stored in an air-tight container.

Makes 14 servings
250 g (9 oz) porridge oats
75 g (3 oz) wholewheat flakes
50 g (2 oz) bran buds
2 tbsp chopped walnuts, hazelnuts, almonds
75 g (3 oz) sunflower seeds
175 g (6 oz) sultanas
175 g (6 oz) dried apricots (or figs, pears or peaches, or a mixture)
Soya milk
Honey or syrup (optional)
Cinnamon (optional)
- Mix together the oats, wholewheat flakes, bran buds, nuts, sunflower seeds and dried fruit and store in an air-tight container until required.
- Pour the desired amount into a bowl and add plenty of soya milk. If desired, add honey or syrup and sprinkle powdered cinnamon over the top.

Country Casserole

Serves 4
450 ml ($^3/4$ pt) water
pinch of salt
150 g (5 oz) buckwheat
30 ml (2 tbsp) vegetable oil
1 red or green pepper, cored, seeded and cut into strips
1 onion, skinned and finely chopped
350 g (12 oz) courgettes, trimmed and sliced
175 g (6 oz) mushrooms, sliced
225 g (8 oz) red split lentils
3 bay leaves
30 ml (2 tbsp) lemon juice
1 garlic clove, skinned and crushed
2 rosemary sprigs
5 ml (1 tsp) cumin seeds
600 ml (1 pt) vegetable stock (or dissolved stock cube in water)
250g (1 oz) low-fat margarine

salt and black pepper
chopped fresh parsley, to garnish
- Bring the water to the boil in a saucepan, add the salt, then sprinkle in the buckwheat and return to the boil. Boil rapidly for 1 minute. Reduce the heat, cover and cook gently for 12 minutes or until the water has been absorbed. Do not stir. Transfer to a buttered covered dish.
- Heat the oil in a pot or flameproof casserole cooker and fry the pepper and onion for 5 minutes. Add the courgettes and mushrooms and fry for 5 minutes. Stir in the lentils, bay leaves, lemon juice, garlic, rosemary, cumin and stock. Add the buckwheat and stir well.
- Simmer for about 45 minutes until the lentils are cooked, stirring occasionally. Add the margarine, adjust the seasoning and sprinkle with parsley. Serve hot with crusty wholegrain bread or brown rice.

Dried Fruit Compote

Serves 6
50 g (2 oz) dried apple rings
50 g (2 oz) dried apricots
50 g (2 oz) dried figs
300 ml ($^1/_2$ pt) unsweetened orange juice
300 ml ($^1/_2$ pt) water
25 g (1 oz) hazelnuts
- Cut the dried apples, apricots and figs into chunky pieces and place in a bowl. Mix together the unsweetened orange juice and water and pour over the fruit in the bowl. Cover and leave to soak in the fridge overnight.
- When ready to serve, spread the hazelnuts out in a grill pan and toast under a low to moderate heat, shaking the pan frequently until the hazelnuts are browned evenly on all sides.
- Tip the hazelnuts into a clean tea-towel and rub them while they are still hot to remove the skins. Chop the hazelnuts roughly using an automatic chopper or large cook's knife. Sprinkle over the compote just before serving.

Chapter Eight

Coping with Stress

Tackling chronic stress is a priority for IBS sufferers - with good reason. Apart from triggering IBS symptoms, chronic stress can lead to a host of other conditions including high blood pressure, heart disease, stroke, gastric ulcers, increased risk of infection and chronic anxiety and depression.

Stress and IBS

Although control of the bowel is modulated mainly via the parasympathetic nervous system, when we are under stress, sympathetic nerves take charge. Among its many effects, the sympathetic system stimulates the enteric system to increase stomach and bowel activity. These organs begin to 'churn', and there is an increase in stomach and bowel secretions.

Even non-IBS sufferers are conscious of this heightened gut activity when stressed, nervous or scared. In IBS sufferers the bowel already over-reacts to routine stimuli, so the increased activity caused by stress can trigger IBS symptoms or make those symptoms much worse.

Common Types of Stressors

The link between work-related stress and IBS symptoms is well established. Many IBS sufferers say their symptoms are worst on Monday mornings (with the prospect of the working week ahead), whereas their best times are Friday nights and Saturday mornings (with the prospect of a weekend off).

Any emotional crisis, however, can be a stressor and trigger IBS symptoms. While the list of potential stressors is endless and of course highly individual, some of the most common ones include:

- bereavement, especially of a partner, close relative or friend
- change of job or work location
- divorce, separation or other relationship breakdown
- imprisonment
- life-changing health event such as the menopause, or major surgery such as a hysterectomy or prostatectomy
- loss of job, through being fired, made redundant or taking retirement

- moving house
- serious illness affecting the IBS sufferer or his or her partner, child or close relative.

Seeking Professional Help

Stressors such as bereavement or relationship difficulties may need the support of trained counsellors or therapists (see Chapter Eleven). Extreme stressors such as violent physical or sexual assault, or the effect of a car crash or rail disaster, either as a victim, rescuer or onlooker, can lead to a condition called post-traumatic stress disorder. This condition, found more often in IBS sufferers than in others, requires specialist medical treatment.

It is beyond the scope of this book to cover all the possible stressors you may encounter and suggest how to manage them. Your doctor will be able to put you in touch with the appropriate health care professional. Many forms of stress, however, can be tackled through changes in mental outlook, lifestyle and behaviour. For example, some of the measures discussed in Chapter Five, such as taking more exercise and developing a more positive attitude, will also greatly improve stress levels.

Managing Stress

The first step to managing stress is to accept that you have a problem. You can then identify those factors that may be contributing to your stress levels and so develop a strategy for dealing with them. The next step is to genuinely want to tackle them.

IBS may be the incentive you need to take a hard look at long-standing problems, and make some changes. This may mean taking difficult decisions - but unless you want your IBS symptoms to continue, you have to accept this fact.

Of course, tackling major life problems is often easier said than done. Stressors are bound to be difficult to deal with - if they weren't they wouldn't cause stress. But perhaps you should think of IBS as a warning bell alerting you to the urgent need to make important life decisions. IBS, although distressing, is not life-threatening. Other stress-related disorders, such as heart disease, most certainly are.

One common cause of chronic stress is simply taking on too much, often because you don't want to let others down. Perhaps you are taking on extra job responsibilities, juggling job and family commitments, doing voluntary work or striving to maintain unrealistic living standards.

Learn to Delegate

If your main problem is that you are doing too much, the answer is to do less. What tasks can you delegate, and what can you give up? You may find that work colleagues or family members would be only too happy to help.

Accept Your Limitations

If the problem stems from the fact that you are living beyond your means, ask yourself why you are trying to maintain such an expensive lifestyle. Is it that you think others might look down on you if you don't drive the latest car, or have expensive foreign holidays?

Ask yourself if these things really matter and, if you decide they don't, look at ways you can economize. Once you discover that you don't actually need to earn so much, you might find you can reduce your workload - and start to enjoy life. You may then find your symptoms improve dramatically.

Hell Is Other People

In many cases, stress arises from a troubled relationship, perhaps with a partner, relative, child, colleague or superior. You may have been trying to ignore the fact that there was a problem in order to avoid confrontation, or because you were unwilling to face up to the cause. If you are serious about tackling your symptoms, perhaps now is the time to accept that the issue must be resolved. The first step is to talk the matter over. Find a time when you can talk to the person calmly and rationally. Try to see things from his or her point of view and avoid confrontation. Be patient and make sure you give the other party plenty of time to speak. You may then be able to suggest a compromise.

You may find that having 'cleared the air', the relationship will have improved dramatically, or that you have resolved the underlying problem. If not, perhaps there is someone who can act as an intermediary, such as a friend, respected family member, or more senior figure in the company.

Ultimately, though, you may need to accept that there is no solution and that definite action is called for. This might mean accepting that a personal relationship is doomed and finishing it for good, asking to be moved to another department at work, or changing jobs. However upsetting this may be in the short term, ultimately your physical health and mental well-being (and your IBS symptoms) should improve as a consequence.

Don't Suffer Alone

The importance of relationships in helping you to deal with stress cannot be underestimated. Close-knit communities, such as religious groups, often have a lower than average incidence of stress symptoms. The sense of belonging, and of being able to turn to others for sympathy and help, are powerful antidotes to stress - and to stress-related IBS symptoms. It is not always necessary to join a religious group to gain these benefits. Just talking things over with friends or relatives can ease the pressure.

You may not realize how much a stressor has been affecting you until you discuss it with someone. Hearing another's point of view can help to put a problem in perspective and help you realize that perhaps it is not as serious as you thought, or, that the time has come to act.

Get a Pet

Countless studies have proved that keeping a pet reduces stress levels and counteracts depression and anxiety. Pet owners have lower blood pressure and reduced blood levels of LDL ('bad') cholesterol, compared with others. As a consequence, they have lower rates of heart disease and strokes. For dog owners who take their charges for regular walks, and hence get plenty of exercise, the difference in health status may be even more marked.

The ABC Approach

Not all forms of stress are avoidable. In some cases the best approach is to change the way you *react* to stressful events. There are methods you can try. One used by cognitive-behavioural therapists (see Chapter Eleven) is the ABC approach. A stands for 'antecedent', B for 'behaviour' and C for 'consequences'.

Think about a particular incident where your reaction to a stressful incident actually made things worse. For example, suppose your journey to work was longer than normal because you got stuck in a traffic jam (*antecedent*), and you sounded your horn and shouted at other drivers (*behaviour*). When you finally got to work, you were bad-tempered with colleagues and found it difficult to concentrate on the task in hand (*consequences*).

Now, review this sequence of events in your mind to see if you could have done anything to change the antecedent, or your behaviour, and so alter the consequences. For example, in future you might:

- allow more time for your journey and take a different (possibly more scenic) route to work
- buy a language tape and learn useful phrases for business or holidays during your journey
- find a practical way to make use of the extra time, perhaps by thinking about the day ahead and planning what you are going to do
- listen to the radio, and sing along loudly
- practise deep breathing to help you to get into a relaxed frame of mind

- think of some other techniques you can use to make the most of the time if you get stuck in another traffic jam, or your train is late or flight delayed.

TakeTime to Uwind

No matter how busy you are, set aside time each day to rest, relax and 'switch off'. Make this 'me' time when your own needs are paramount. Use the time to do something you enjoy, like reading, listening to music or practising a hobby such as painting or collecting. It is also worth while learning a relaxation technique which you can use to make your 'me' time more therapeutic. Practise a technique you can use to stay calm whenever you feel tense, anxious and pressured, for example at work. There are many kinds. But they all have two main aims - to relax the muscles and calm the mind.

Choose a time when you know you'll be free from distractions. Find a part of the house that you associate with calm, such as a lounge or bedroom, and make yourself comfortable on a chair or on a cushion on the floor.

It is a good idea to place a favourite picture, photograph or ornament nearby that is small enough to fit into your bag or pocket. This will be your 'symbol of calm'. After a while you will find that, wherever you are, whenever you feel tense, you'll be able to look at your symbol and instantly relax.

Deep Breathing

This is one of the most effective relaxation techniques. You can use this at home, work, when travelling, or any time you need to ease tension. Deep breathing can be used on its own or in combination with other techniques such as meditation, visualization and progressive muscular relaxation (see below).

When you are tense your breathing tends to be fast but shallow. When you are calm you tend to take deep, slow breaths. So, to reduce your tension change your breathing pattern: breathe deeply, from the diaphragm (the sheet of muscle that separates your lungs from your abdomen) rather than from the tops of the lungs, when you use just your chest muscles.

Lie on the floor with one hand on your chest and the other on your abdomen. Breathe slowly through your nose, taking the air deep down into your abdomen. Hold the breath for a while and then let it out slowly.

If you are breathing correctly, you should feel the hand on your abdomen rise and fall, while the other hand hardly moves at all. Once you have mastered this method of breathing, you should aim to use it all the time - sitting, standing, wherever you are - not just as an aid to relaxation.

Meditation

This technique calms the mind. Focus on your breathing, an abstract image, a candle flame, or a single word or sound that you repeat softly to yourself. Breathe deeply from your abdomen and feel the tension draining out of you and passing into the floor. Take as long as you like. When you finish, take a few moments to keep perfectly still and enjoy the feeling of serenity.

One easy form of meditation to try is breath-counting (a technique known to Zen Buddhists as *za-zen* or 'sitting meditation'). Use the deep breathing technique you have been practising, but count your breaths in cycles of 10.

Breathe slowly and count the in-breaths only. Each time you reach 10, start again. Concentrate on nothing but counting. If another thought starts to intrude, acknowledge it, tell yourself you will return to the thought later, and then go back to breath-counting.

Deep Muscle Relaxation (DMR)

This is a way of ridding your body of tension that has built up during the day.

1. Lie flat on your back with your legs a little way apart and your hands away from your body, palms facing up.
2. Close your eyes and focus on your breathing. Breathe deeply, using the diaphragmatic technique you have already practised, and concentrate on your breath flowing smoothly in and out of your body.
3. Mentally seek out areas of tension. Each time you exhale, imagine that the tension is floating away. Pay particular attention to your face, jaw, neck, shoulders and back - areas where a build-up of tension is common.
4. Feel your body sink into the floor. Focus on each set of muscles in turn, starting with the feet and working your way up your body. Feel your muscles getting weak and heavy. Imagine your body is no longer a part of you and simply let it lie there unmoving.

Progressive Muscular Relaxation

This is a similar technique to DMR, and involves tensing and then relaxing your muscles in turn, starting at your feet.

1. Tense the muscles for 5 seconds before relaxing them. As you do so, concentrate on the sense of warmth and heaviness you feel. First, clench your toes and point your feet to tense your calf muscles. Hold for 5 seconds and then release.
2. Work up the body, tightening first the thigh muscles, then the buttocks and abdomen. Clench and relax your hands, tense and release your arms and shoulders.

3. To finish, screw up your face, then open your mouth and eyes wide and release them. Now lie still and concentrate on your breathing.

Clear Your Mind

You will probably find that having a stressful day leaves you tense, irritable or even angry, and unable to relax. It may stop you getting to sleep. Any relaxation method you attempt may fail unless you can clear your mind of the jumble of anxious thoughts you are left with at the end of the day.

Try writing your worries down as a list. Now make a separate column marked 'to do' and list the actions you need to take to deal 'with those problems'. If you haven't come up with a solution, simply put 'think about it some more.' Re-write your list and place each item in order of priority. Once you are satisfied that you have externalized your problems by getting them down on paper, you'll find it easier to put them into perspective.

Visualization to Clear Your Mind

Unlike meditation, which empties the mind of all thought, visualization is designed to replace anxious thoughts with restful images.

Find a quiet place where you can sit still and quietly review the day in your mind. You may find there are key moments that stand out - an unpleasant incident, say, or a hurtful remark.

Now see yourself blowing bubbles, as you did as a child. Imagine each irksome moment is a bubble. It drifts up and away on the wind, slowly getting smaller until it vanishes from sight. Do this with each irritation in turn, until they have all gone.

Pack Up Your Troubles

Perhaps there is a particular event coming up that is worrying you, such as an examination or an appraisal, and it is making you tense. You can use visualization here, too. Once you have made sure you are fully prepared for the event and there is nothing else practical that you can do, 'pack it away' in your mind and forget about it for a while. This is how you do it:

Think of an item that can represent the event that worries you. For an exam, you could think of a reference book; for an appraisal, imagine a folder. Now visualize yourself putting the item away into a secure filing cabinet.

See yourself opening the drawer of the filing cabinet. Pick up the book or folder and place it in the bottom of the drawer. Close the drawer firmly and lock it. Now, imagine yourself turning away from the filing cabinet and walking from the room. You can return to that cabinet and retrieve the item any time you want, but for now it is 'out of sight' and you can forget it.

Using Calming Images

You can also use visualization techniques to calm your mind. Think of a relaxing scene. It could be imaginary or drawn from memory. Perhaps it is a pretty grass-covered hill overlooking beautiful woodland, a sun-drenched beach on a tropical island, or a cool mountain stream that sparkles as it tumbles over rocks.

You may find a domestic scene more relaxing, such as the front parlour in the home of a favourite aunt whom you would visit as a child, or a favourite picture in an art gallery that you like to visit.

Invest the scene with as much detail as possible. For example, if you are picturing a woodland glade, see yourself stretched out on the grass. Smell the grass, plants and flowers all around, feel the soft breeze and the warmth of the sun on your skin. Imagine the blue sky above you with fluffy white clouds drifting lazily along. Try to make the image as realistic as possible, so that you can call it to mind whenever you need its calming influence.

Picture the Scene

If you have difficulty visualizing a suitable image, another technique is to look at a restful painting, print or photograph, or an illustration in a book or magazine. Study the picture for several minutes, looking at it in detail. Judge the colours, the composition and the skill that went into producing it.

Now close your eyes and try to keep the image in mind. Remember as many details as you can. Look at the picture again. Is it as you remember it? Check whether you forgot any details or are seeing something new.

Sleep Well

Many people find that they have disturbed sleep or sleepless nights when under stress. In fact, stress and sleeplessness (insomnia) go hand in hand. Stress makes it difficult to get to sleep, and lack of sleep makes you more stressed. There are steps you can take to tackle this problem.

Reserve the hour or so before you go to bed for relaxing pursuits, such as reading a book (ideally, a boring one or one you know well and so will not be tempted to stay awake to finish).

Avoid eating a large meal too close to bedtime. Instead, have a glass of soya milk and eat some almonds or peanuts with a biscuit, or a banana. Soya, almonds and peanuts contain the amino acid tryptophan, used to make the brain chemicals melatonin and serotonin that are needed to regulate sleep. Tryptophan is absorbed into the brain more efficiently if there is plenty of carbohydrate present.

Don't stimulate your mind or body too close to bedtime. Avoid playing sport, or doing keep-fit exercises or watching an exciting television programme just before you go to bed. And don't have caffeinated drinks such as coffee, tea or some colas, within six hours of bedtime.

If you find it difficult to get to sleep, get out of bed and sit in a chair until you start to feel sleepy again. It might help to get out that boring book again, or write a letter. Don't just lie in bed feeling anxious about the fact that sleep won't come. Otherwise your subconscious can start to associate bed with anxiety about getting to sleep. You will then feel anxious and wide awake whenever you are lying in bed, even when you are not stressed.

Calming Jumbled Thoughts

You can adapt some of the visualization and other relaxation tips already mentioned. If you can't get to sleep because your head is full of jumbled thoughts, think of an image to still your mind. For example, imagine you have swept your thoughts into a heap - like a big pile of leaves. Listen as a gentle breeze springs up and starts to blow the leaves away, first in small flurries and then in ones and twos, until the leaves are gone and all is still.

Alternatively, you might see yourself on the deck of a ship sailing across a stormy ocean. Your chaotic thoughts are the huge waves crashing against the side of the sturdy vessel. Listen to the noise of the wind and waves, and feel the salt spray against your face. Now, gradually let the waves grow calmer. Listen as the sound of the wind and waves gradually recedes. Finally, imagine the sun glinting off a perfectly flat ocean. With practice and patience, you should find an image that works best for you.

Many of the relaxation methods described in this chapter can also help you to manage painful IBS symptoms - and there are many other tips and techniques you can try. Pain-management is tackled in the next chapter.

Case Study: Sonia
Sonia has found that stress management has made a big difference to her symptoms: 'When the pain has been very bad I have had to take a week off work. I find just sitting down doing nothing can work wonders. Of course, you can't always just take a break from work. But even when I am at work, if I can take five minutes out to relax it really helps. I'm getting quite good at stress management. What keeps me calm and puts a big smile on my face and just relaxes me are pictures of my friends and family. I've got pictures that I carry around with me, everywhere I go. I can just take them out and look at them at any time. At home, I've got loads of pictures of friends and family that I've placed all around the house. That's one thing that always works for me. When I'm feeling stressed I just look at my pictures and I feel fine.'

Chapter Nine

Pain-management

The simplest way to manage pain is to use painkillers. Paracetamol (US name, acetaminophen) is a mild and effective painkiller for symptoms such as abdominal pain (and menstrual pain, which can trigger IBS symptoms). It is safe for most people, provided you don't exceed the dosage (see Chapter Ten).

Paracetamol blocks the signals travelling along pain pathways in the central nervous system. IBS is not an inflammatory disorder, so paracetamol may be more effective than aspirin, which blocks the action of prostaglandins, chemicals that cause the pain, reddening and swelling of inflammation.

Your doctor may prescribe different painkillers, or other medications with a painkilling effect, such as antispasmodics (see Chapter Ten). Some people prefer complementary medicines, such as herbal remedies (see Chapter Twelve).

For chronic conditions such as IBS, drugs can offer only short-term relief, whenever symptoms are particularly severe. Some painkillers may even become less effective if used for long periods. A more effective approach may be to understand pain perception (see Chapter Three), and use this information to develop self-help measures that can alleviate your pain or reduce it to manageable levels.

Pain Tolerance

Your reaction to pain - all forms, not just the pain of IBS - is not a simple matter but a response that has been developed over time and is influenced by many factors, including your emotional state.

Everyone has their pain threshold. In general, women can tolerate somatic pain (affecting the skin, bones and muscles) much better than men, but have a lower tolerance to visceral pain (affecting the internal organs). But there is little difference between men and women in overall pain tolerance.

Our personal pain threshold also varies according to heredity, upbringing, cultural background, age and previous experiences. For example, pain may be particularly distressing to a younger person who has never experienced anything like it before and who is understandably anxious.

Older people may be more tolerant of a similar level of pain as they can draw on past experiences to help them cope. They may know, for example, what is causing the pain and how long it is likely to last. They remember how they coped with the pain before and so are more confident they can bear it this time.

Emotional Factors

Anxiety can make you more sensitive to a painful experience, whereas excitement can increase your pain threshold. This was first discovered by Dr Henry K. Beecher, Professor of Anaesthetics at Harvard University, when he was treating soldiers during the Second World War. He noticed that soldiers needed less pain relief than civilians who had suffered similar injuries.

His conclusion was that our experience of pain depends on our emotional state at the time of the injury. For soldiers, caught up in the adrenalin rush of war, a minor wound may be ignored until more immediate dangers have passed. Also, they were prepared for the possibility of injury, and even badly wounded soldiers took comfort from the fact that things could be worse - they could be dead.

Civilians, on the other hand, viewed pain differently. The injury was, in all likelihood, unexpected and so they not only felt shocked that they had been wounded, but also a sense of injustice, which made them depressed. Consequently, they felt pain more keenly and required more pain relief.

One theory for this is that your mental state influences the levels of natural painkillers (endorphins) your body produces, and hence the level of pain you experience. Positive mental states, such as being relaxed, happy and optimistic - mediated by the emotional motor system (EMS) - stimulate endorphin release, whereas negative mental states such as anxiety and depression tend to inhibit its release.

Anxiety can heighten all your senses, not just pain perception. This may be a throwback to earlier times when humans had to be extra vigilant in unfamiliar territory, in case of attack from wild animals or hostile invaders.

When you are tense you will find that noises seem louder and that you are more aware of movement and smells, and more easily startled. IBS sufferers are already hypersensitive to signals emanating from their bowel, so this heightened awareness may make abdominal pain seem far worse.

Stressful events not only trigger IBS symptoms via the stress response (see Chapter Eight) but also heighten your perception of pain via the close link between your pain centres and the limbic centre (the seat of your emotional responses), again mediated by the EMS.

A relationship breakdown, for example, causes initial feelings of rejection, betrayal, anger and hurt, followed by anxiety and depression. The stress of the breakdown triggers your IBS symptoms, and your emotional state makes the pain you experience seem even worse. This leads to a vicious circle in which your mental state disturbs your sleep pattern, giving you restless nights. You awake feeling tired and irritable, which affects your work performance and relationships with friends and colleagues. This increases your stress levels and exacerbates the pain of IBS.

Finding a Coping Strategy

IBS sufferers - indeed everyone - probably experiences pain in their own unique way. So, to manage pain you may need to find a strategy, or more likely a combination of strategies, that is personal to you. Many of the techniques already covered in this book, such as positive affirmations (Chapter Five) and relaxation methods (Chapter Eight) can help you manage pain.

Some forms of complementary therapy, such as acupuncture, have also proved effective for many people, probably by raising endorphin levels (see ChapterTwelve). There are also other approaches you may find useful.

Overcoming Fear

Fear of IBS can make your condition seem far worse. If you talk to your doctor and learn as much about IBS as you can, this may put your mind at rest. You could speak to other sufferers to learn from their experiences and perhaps pick up useful tips. By demystifying the symptoms you'll have gone a long way to easing your fears - and hence bringing the pain and other symptoms under control.

Dealing with Emotional Pain

The way you deal with emotional hurts can also reduce IBS-related pain. Instead of repressing your fears, anxieties and frustrations, discuss your emotions openly with friends and relatives. Try to focus on the positive aspects of your life rather than dwelling on negative ones, and challenge any unhelpful automatic responses to pain that you might make. For example, if you find yourself saying, 'I can't bear this any more', remind yourself that you coped yesterday and tell yourself you will cope even better today.

Helping Others

There is plenty of evidence to show that helping those who are worse off can make us feel better. This is partly because activity offers an important distraction, but also because it helps to improve self-esteem. You could visit elderly or housebound relatives or neighbours for a chat, or offer practical help such as taking their dog for a walk or doing their shopping.

Be prepared to accept help from others, too. When your IBS symptoms are getting you down it is easy to cut yourself off and try to carry on by yourself. But this may be seen as rejection by friends or relatives, who genuinely want to do something for you. By encouraging their support, you strengthen the relationship and increase your feelings of self-worth and of being wanted.

Distracting Yourself

When you are suffering pain you may limit activities for fear of making it worse. But this makes you focus on the pain more strongly. You will reduce your perception of pain if you can distract yourself by keeping occupied.

There may be some simple tasks that you have been putting off which you can do. Taking up a hobby, pastime or looking through old letters, diaries and photographs can help take your mind off painful symptoms.

Using Laughter
You probably don't feel much like laughing when you are in pain. Yet it can be a great antidote. 'Laughter is the best medicine' is almost literally true when it comes to pain-management. A belly laugh, a chuckle, or just a smile of wry amusement is thought to stimulate the release of mood-enhancing brain chemicals and activate the body's various pain-relief mechanisms.

Laughter is also a well-tried method of distraction. Always keep at hand a favourite book or tape of a comedy film, television or radio show that you know always makes you laugh.

The Power of Touch
Rubbing or massaging your abdomen can help ease the griping pain of IBS (see Chapter Twelve). This 'closes' the pain gate and prevents pain signals from reaching the brain. But you can also block pain signals with heat therapy:

Soak a small towel or large handkerchief in hot water. Wring it out and then fold it to a convenient size and press it against the painful area of your abdomen. You may need to repeat this from time to time until the pain passes. A hot water bottle or an electric blanket can also be effective.

Visualization for Pain Relief
This technique is not only useful for stress relief, it can also help alleviate abdominal pain. One theory is that visualization stimulates activity in the

descending anti-pain nerve pathways which block pain signals. The following examples show how the technique is used in pain-management. But you will probably think of a visualization that works better for you.

You may need to experiment with a variety of images, and practise them several times before you notice the benefit. To make your visualizations more effective, choose images that match the kind of pain you feel and the sort of sensation you imagine would bring relief. For example:

- For burning pain, you might visualize a fire burning in the middle of a lush, green forest. Now imagine the sky filling with shiny rain clouds. Picture cooling rain falling on to the fire and quelling the flames - you can even see steam rising from the flames. As the rain falls more heavily the fire will begin to shrink. As the fire diminishes, you will feel the pain recede until only a few glowing embers are left. As they vanish, so does your pain.
- For a gnawing pain, you might visualize a huge shark swimming in the depths of a vast ocean. Now imagine that a group of dolphins has arrived and is circling the shark. More and more dolphins appear to surround the beast and force it further and further from you. As the fleeing shark shrinks to a tiny dot in the distance, feel the pain ebb away. Once the shark vanishes from sight, your pain will have gone too.
- For stabbing pain, visualize a long, sharp piece of ice digging into your abdomen. Now imagine you are sitting in front of a warm fire. As the heat from the flames grows stronger, feel the ice begin to melt. As the ice shrinks, your pain diminishes. Soon there is little left of the ice but a small pool of water. Then this too is gone - along with your pain.

Setting Goals

Overcoming any chronic pain condition is a psychological battle. It is all too easy to lose heart. One way to stay optimistic is to set yourself realistic goals so that you know you are making progress. This is called 'pain-pacing'.

If a painful attack normally causes you to take to your bed and remain there for the next hour, try to cope by sitting in a chair instead, perhaps with a pillow or hot water bottle against your abdomen.

Once you have managed that goal on several occasions, next time try to avoid sitting down and, instead, carry out a few simple tasks or take a short walk, to help take your mind off the pain. Over the following days or weeks, plan more ambitious targets. By setting goals, and reaching them, you gain the confidence to continue - each time setting your sights a little higher.

There may be times when you do not make the progress you hoped for.

This is only natural. But by concentrating on the overall progress you're making, and continuing to stretch yourself, you'll find that the pain has less impact on your life. When carried out in conjunction with other measures, such as relaxation techniques, pain-pacing can help you regain control of your life.

You may find self-help measures alone cannot adequately control your IBS symptoms, and that professional help is necessary. This is dealt with in Part 3.

Part Three

Treating IBS

Chapter Ten

Medications for IBS

There are numerous drugs available to alleviate IBS symptoms. Many can be bought over the counter at the pharmacist's, but these can give rather limited results. More effective medicines may be prescribed by your doctor.

As there is no 'cure' for IBS, the main aim of drug treatment is to stabilize your condition and improve your quality of life, so allowing time for self-help strategies (such as dietary changes and stress- and pain-management) to be effective. Ideally, the drug treatment can then be phased out.

There is no standard drug treatment for IBS. Sufferers are considered the most important 'clinicians' in determining their own treatment, so you will need to work with your doctor to find the most effective drug regime. This may involve a degree of trial and error.

Drugs for Physical Symptoms

There are three main categories of drug used in IBS: laxatives, to encourage bowel movement; antidiarrhoeals, to make the stool firmer and reduce the sensation of urgency; and antispasmodics/smooth muscle relaxants, to prevent muscle spasms. There are also other drugs for symptoms such as pain, flatulence and heartburn.

Laxatives

Many kinds of laxative are available over the counter from pharmacies. These should be used as a short-term measure only. If your constipation persists, see your doctor, who may suggest you try a different type of laxative, or prescribe a drug that is not available over the counter.

Laxatives come in many forms: as a food supplement, powder, granules, tablets or capsules. In severe cases, patients may be treated with enemas or suppositories. Although laxatives are mainly for people with constipation-predominant or alternating IBS, they may be prescribed to those suffering from diarrhoea-predominant IBS, to help regulate bowel movement. There are four main types of laxative: bulk-forming, osmotic, stimulant, and faecal softeners.

Bulk-forming Laxatives

Ideally, you should increase your fibre intake through dietary means, simply by eating more naturally fibre-rich foods. However, as a short-term measure you may choose to take bulk-forming laxatives. There are several kinds, but all work in much the same ways, by absorbing water and increasing in size, thereby stimulating bowel activity. It may take a few days for bulk-forming laxatives to work, so don't expect instant results.

The most common types are unprocessed wheat bran or oat bran. Bran can come as a coarse powder which is sprinkled over food, or eaten as bran bread or bran biscuits, or taken in tablet form. You must then drink plenty of water or fruit juice with the meal to help the bran to swell. Finely ground bran, especially in bread or biscuits, is more palatable than less processed types, but not so effective at absorbing water.

The fibre in bulk-forming laxatives can hinder the absorption of important vitamins and minerals, so always maintain a healthy, balanced diet to avoid a deficiency of these nutrients.

It is vitally important that you drink plenty of fluids - especially, but not only, at mealtimes - or you may make your constipation much worse. In extreme cases your bowel can get blocked - a potentially serious condition.

Initially, some bulk-forming laxatives may exacerbate IBS symptoms such as flatulence, until the bowel adjusts to the change. So start with a small quantity and slowly increase the amount. For example, in the case of bran tablets, have one per meal, three times a day, and gradually increase to three per meal as necessary.

For people who cannot tolerate bran there are other bulk-forming laxatives, such as corn fibre (often eaten as a biscuit), ispaghula husk, sterculia and methylcellulose (which also has the property of softening stools to make them easier to pass).

Osmotic Laxatives

The main function of an osmotic laxative is to retain water in the bowel and so soften the stool. The most widely used are mineral salts, such as Epsom salts (magnesium sulphate), magnesium citrate and magnesium hydroxide.

Substances such as lactulose, lactitol and sorbitol-sugars act as both osmotic and bulk-forming laxatives because they help retain water and increase in size. As with other bulk-forming laxatives, it is vital to drink plenty of water when using these medicines.

Stimulant Laxatives

These drugs stimulate bowel movement, in some cases by irritating the bowel lining. They are powerful and so should only be used under medical supervision, and then only in severe cases. They can cause stomach cramps, and there is a risk that they may affect bowel function adversely, especially if used over long periods. They include bisacodyl and docusate sodium.

There are other stimulant laxatives available over the counter, in various unstandardized compound formulations, which should be avoided in IBS because their action is too drastic and unpredictable. These include aloes, cascara, colocynth, frangula, rhubarb and senna.

Faecal Softeners

These are used in severe cases of constipation and, as the name suggests, are designed to soften hardened and compacted stools. The two most common types are liquid paraffin, taken orally, and arachis (peanut) oil, used as an enema.

Antidiarrhoeals

Also called antimotility drugs, antidiarrhoeals may be effective for people with D-IBS or A-IBS. Common antidiarrhoeals include loperamide hydrochloride and codeine phosphate. Loperamide is available over the counter. Others are available only on prescription.

Antidiarrhoeals known as adsorbent drugs (kaolin, and kaolin/morphine mixtures, for example) may not be suitable for chronic conditions such as IBS (an exception is aluminium hydroxide when used in a compound medicine - see page 91).

Antispasmodics

These drugs relax the smooth muscle of the bowel wall and so prevent the muscular spasms that cause pain, bloating, constipation and/or diarrhoea. This group includes the antimuscarinics (or anticholinergics) such as atropine sulphate, dicloverine/dicyclomine hydrochloride, hyoscine butylbromide, and propantheline bromide.

Other antispasmodics, known as smooth muscle relaxants, include alverine citrate, mebeverine hydrochloride and peppermint oil. (In studies, peppermint oil proved effective in relieving the abdominal pain and bloating of IBS, particularly in children. However, it can cause digestive upsets in people who are sensitive to menthol.) You should check with your doctor before taking smooth muscle relaxants if you are suffering from kidney or other bowel disorders, or are pregnant or breastfeeding.

Compound Medicines

Compound medicines contain more than one active ingredient, most commonly an antispasmodic combined with a bulk-forming laxative or an antidiarrhoeal. Common laxative compounds include ispaghula husk combined with either propantheline, mebeverine or metronidazole, and sterculia combined with alverine citrate. Common antidiarrhoeal compounds include dicloverine/dicyclomine hydrochloride, combined with aluminium hydroxide and dimeticone/simethicone.

Other Medicines

Activated charcoal, defoaming agents and paracetamol may be helpful too. Activated charcoal is available from pharmacies. It is usually taken to ease dyspepsia, but may relieve distension and excess wind. Defoaming agents (surfactants) such as dimeticone/simethicone can ease colicky pain and wind.

Paracetamol is a relatively safe painkiller for mild to moderate abdominal and menstrual pain. It can be used in compound drugs along with codeine (an opioid analgesic). Caffeine may be included too, to counteract codeine's sedative effect. As caffeine aggravates IBS symptoms, and may exacerbate pain, compounds containing caffeine are best avoided.

Side-effects

Many of the drugs taken for IBS have potential side-effects. Not everyone will experience them, and even if they do occur they are usually mild. However, if you notice any unusual or unpleasant symptoms after taking a medicine, tell your doctor.

If you suffer serious side-effects such as severe abdominal pain, breathlessness, confusion, dizziness, nausea, rash or vomiting, you should stop taking the medicine and call your doctor. Always follow your doctor's advice when taking medication, and read the instructions and warnings printed on the side of the packet or in any accompanying literature.

Psychotropic Drugs

Your doctor may also prescribe low doses of psychotropic drugs, such as sedatives/tranquillizers or antidepressants. These drugs can help in two ways. First, some psychotropics target chemicals that are active in the bowel as well as the brain. So they not only treat psychological conditions but also alleviate bowel symptoms. Secondly, people with IBS may suffer some degree of anxiety or depression. These patients may benefit from the antidepressant or sedative effect of psychotropic drugs. In most cases, lower doses of antidepressant or sedative are needed for IBS than are given for clinical anxiety or depression. Psychotropic drugs can also act as painkillers - mainly through the close link between mental/emotional state and pain perception.

The terms 'tranquillizer' or 'sedative' cover a large group of drugs. The ones described in this chapter are regularly prescribed in IBS because of their dual brain/bowel action and lower risk of side-effects. However, other tranquillizers may be prescribed, depending on your symptoms.

Antidepressants

Drugs called selective serotonin re-uptake inhibitors (SSRIs) can be effective in treating depression, and are also used to help regulate bowel movement and alleviate pain. Serotonin receptors in the bowel are the target for a new range of drug treatments currently being developed (see below).

Other types of antidepressant, such as the tricyclics, may be used. Low doses of tricyclic antidepressants (imipramine, for example) have been shown to produce significant improvement in patients' IBS symptoms and overall well-being. This may be because these drugs, like the SSRIs, target specific receptors in the bowel, where the sensations that trigger IBS symptoms arise, and in the central nervous system, where these stimuli are processed.

New Drugs

A new generation of drugs, which act at chemical receptor sites in the bowel, are currently undergoing clinical trials and may become available over the coming months or years. There are two general types: agonists, which slot into receptor sites and mimic the effect of a given chemical, and antagonists, which block and inhibit a body chemical's effect. Depending on which receptors are targeted by a drug, it should be possible to increase bowel movement to relieve constipation, or reduce bowel movement to relieve diarrhoea, as well as treating symptoms such as muscle spasms, pain and bloating.

For example, many new drugs target serotonin receptors in the bowel. Serotonin is also known as 5-hydroxytryptamine - or 5-HT, for short. Some 14 types of serotonin receptor have so far been identified - of which 5-HT1, 5-HT3 and 5-HT4 seem most useful for drug therapy. These receptors are, in effect, 'on' and 'off' buttons. The 5-HT4 receptors act as 'on' buttons, stimulating increased bowel motility, whereas the 5-HT3 receptors have the opposite effect. Receptor 5-HT4 may also be involved in the regulation of gut sensitivity and the perception of pain and discomfort. The most important drugs tested so far are cilansetron and ondansetron (5-HT3 antagonists), and tegaserod and prucalopride (5-HT4 agonists).

Ondansetron is primarily used in the treatment of nausea and vertigo. However, in clinical trials it has also had some effect in treating D-IBS, including symptoms of abdominal pain and distension.

In clinical trials, tegaserod proved effective in treating women with C-IBS. Patients showed significant improvements in bowel function, abdominal pain and discomfort, bloating and overall well-being. Adverse effects such as nausea, headache and diarrhoea were noted in a few patients. Prucalopride has proved successful in treating chronic constipation (in some patients), and had some effect on pain and bloating, as well. It may be useful in IBS patients who do not respond to other laxatives.

Drugs Used to Treat IBS

The following chart shows the main drugs used to treat IBS symptoms. All medicines are listed by their generic name, not their brand name (which may vary according to the company producing the drug and the country in which it is available).

Before you buy a remedy over the counter, ask the pharmacist which one may be best for you. Be sure to give any information about your symptoms, general health and medical history that may be relevant. Always consult a doctor before buying over-the-counter drugs for children, the elderly, pregnant or breastfeeding women and anyone with serious, on-going health problems.

Although some medications prescribed for IBS may alleviate psychological symptoms, for some patients counselling or some other form of psychological treatment may be beneficial, too. This subject is covered in the next chapter.

Please see over for chart.

Bulk-forming Laxatives

Bran

How taken:	tablets, powder, bread, biscuits, compound
Availability:	over the counter
Action:	swells when taken with water or other drink to increase stool bulk, stimulate bowel movement and so alleviate constipation
Possible side-effects:	abdominal distension, bowel blockage, flatulence, hypersensitivity
Comments:	consume with a large glass of liquid; maintain adequate fluid intake throughout the course of treatment; do not take close to bedtime

Ispaghula Husk

How taken:	granules, powder, compound
Availability:	over the counter
Action:	swells when taken with water or other drink to increase stool bulk, stimulate bowel movement and so alleviate constipation
Possible side-effects:	abdominal distension, bowel blockage, flatulence, hypersensitivity
Comments:	consume with a large glass of liquid; maintain adequate fluid intake throughout the course of treatment; do not take close to bedtime

Methylcellulose

How taken:	tablets
Availability:	over the counter
Action:	swells when taken with water or other drink to increase stool bulk, stimulate bowel movement and so alleviate constipation
Possible side-effects:	abdominal distension, bowel blockage, flatulence, hypersensitivity
Comments:	consume with a large glass of liquid; maintain adequate fluid intake throughout the course of treatment; do not take close to bedtime

Sterculia

How taken:	granules
Availability:	over the counter
Action:	swells when taken with water or other drink to increase stool bulk, stimulate bowel movement and so alleviate constipation
Possible side-effects:	abdominal distension, bowel blockage, flatulence, hypersensitivity
Comments:	consume with a large glass of liquid; maintain adequate fluid intake throughout the course of treatment; do not take close to bedtime

Stimulant Laxatives

Bisacodyl

How taken:	tablets, suppositories
Availability:	prescription only
Action:	increases intestinal movement to alleviate constipation
Possible side-effects:	abdominal cramps (common), anal irritation (suppositories only)
Comments:	prolonged use can lead to a non-functioning bowel

Docusate Sodium

How taken:	capsules, liquid, suppositories, enema
Availability:	prescription only
Action:	increases intestinal movement to alleviate constipation
Possible side-effects:	abdominal cramps (common)
Comments:	prolonged use can lead to a non-functioning bowel

Glycerin

How taken:	suppositories
Availability:	over the counter
Action:	irritant, stimulates bowel movement and so alleviates constipation
Possible side-effects:	none reported
Comments:	moisten with water before using

Osmotic Laxatives

Lactitol/Lactulose

How taken:	powder (mixed with food), liquid
Availability:	over the counter
Action:	non-digestible sugar that retains water in the bowel, so producing loose faeces, stimulating bowel movement and alleviating constipation
Possible side-effects:	abdominal discomfort or pain, flatulence
Comments:	adequate fluid intake must be maintained throughout the course of treatment

Magnesium hydroxide

How taken:	powder (mixed with food), liquid, compound
Availability:	prescription only
Action:	retains water in the bowel, so producing loose faeces and alleviating constipation
Possible side-effects:	abdominal discomfort or pain
Comments:	for occasional use; maintain adequate fluid intake

Faecal Softeners

Arachis (peanut) Oil

How taken:	enema
Availability:	prescription only
Action:	softens hardened faeces to aid bowel movement and alleviate constipation
Possible side-effects:	allergic reaction
Comments:	not suitable for those with nut allergy

Liquid Paraffin

How taken:	liquid
Availability:	over the counter
Action:	softens hardened faeces to aid bowel movement and alleviate constipation
Possible side-effects:	seepage from anus, irritation, lung and skin disorders, malabsorption of fat-soluble vitamins
Comments:	do not take close to bedtime

Antidiarrhoeals

Codeine phosphate

How taken:	tablets, liquid
Availability:	prescription only
Action:	acts via the central nervous system to reduce bowel movement and so alleviate chronic diarrhoea
Possible side-effects:	breathing difficulties, constipation, drowsiness, nausea
Comments:	generally best avoided, especially for prolonged use, as may cause dependence

Co-phenotrope (diphenoxylate and atropine sulphate)

How taken:	tablets
Availability:	prescription only
Action:	acts via the central nervous system to reduce bowel movement and so alleviate chronic diarrhoea
Possible side-effects:	breathing difficulties, constipation, drowsiness, nausea; possible atropine side-effects in hypersensitive people (see Atropine sulphate, below)
Comments:	generally best avoided, especially for prolonged use, as may cause dependence

Loperamide hydrochloride

How taken:	*tablets, syrup, compound*
Availability:	*over the counter*
Action:	*acts directly on the smooth muscle of the bowel to reduce movement and so alleviate chronic diarrhoea*
Possible side-effects:	*abdominal bloating, abdominal cramps, dizziness, drowsiness and rash*
Comments:	*maintain adequate fluid intake*

Morphine

How taken:	*compound*
Availability:	*prescription only*
Action:	*acts via the central nervous system to reduce bowel movement and so alleviate chronic diarrhoea*
Possible side-effects:	*breathing difficulties, constipation, drowsiness, nausea*
Comments:	*generally best avoided, especially for prolonged use, as may cause dependence*

Antispasmodics

Atropine sulphate

How taken:	*tablets*
Availability:	*prescription only (tablets), over-the-counter (compound)*
Action:	*reduces spasms and bowel motility, relieves pain and diarrhoea. Also effective for dyspepsia (heartburn, bloating and nausea)*
Possible side-effects:	*constipation, dry mouth, dry skin, flushing, irregular heart rate (arrhythmia), rapid heart rate (tachycardia), sensitivity to light (photophobia), slow heart rate (bradycardia), urinary problems, visual problems; (rarely) confusion, giddiness, nausea and vomiting*

Dicloverine/ dicyclomine hydrochloride

How taken:	*tablets, compound*
Availability:	*prescription only (tablets), over the counter (compound)*
Action:	*reduces spasms and bowel movement, relieves pain and diarrhoea. Also effective for dyspepsia (heartburn, bloating and nausea)* *cont...*

Possible side-effects:	constipation, dry mouth, dry skin, flushing, irregular heart rate (arrhythmia), rapid heart rate (tachycardia), sensitivity to light (photophobia), slow heart rate (bradycardia), urinary problems, visual problems; (rarely) confusion, giddiness, nausea and vomiting

Hyoscine buytlbromide

How taken:	tablets
Availability:	prescription only
Action:	reduces spasms and bowel movement, relieves pain and diarrhoea. Also effective for dyspepsia (heartburn, bloating and nausea)
Possible side-effects:	constipation, dry mouth, dry skin, flushing, irregular heart rate (arrhythmia), rapid heart rate (tachycardia), sensitivity to light (photophobia), slow heart rate (bradycardia), urinary problems, visual problems; (rarely) confusion, giddiness, nausea and vomiting

Propantheline bromide

How taken:	tablets
Availability:	prescription only
Action:	reduces spasms and bowel movement, relieves pain and diarrhoea. Also effective against dyspepsia (heartburn, bloating and nausea).
Possible side-effects:	constipation, dry mouth, dry skin, flushing, irregular heart rate (arrhythmia), rapid heart rate (tachycardia), sensitivity to light (photophobia), slow heart rate (bradycardia), urinary problems, visual problems; (rarely) confusion, giddiness, nausea and vomiting

Alverine citrate

How taken:	capsules, compound
Availability:	prescription only
Action:	acts directly to relax the smooth muscle of the bowel to reduce spasms and ease abdominal pain
Possible side-effects:	dizziness, headache, itching (pruritus), nausea and rash
Comments:	as compound medicine, consume with a large glass of liquid; maintain adequate fluid intake throughout the treatment; do not take close to bedtime

Mebeverine hydrochloride

How taken:	tablets, liquid, capsule, compound
Availability:	prescription only
Action:	acts directly to relax the smooth muscle of the bowel to reduce spasms and ease abdominal pain
Possible side-effects:	no serious effects
Comments:	when taken as a compound medicine, consume with a large glass of liquid; maintain adequate fluid intake throughout the treatment; do not take close to bedtime

Peppermint oil

How taken:	capsule
Availability:	over the counter
Action:	acts directly to relax the smooth muscle of the bowel to reduce spasms and relieve abdominal pain, bloating and distension
Possible side-effects:	heartburn and irritation of the anal area; (rarely) allergic reaction, headache, impaired co-ordination (ataxia), muscle tremor, rash and slow heart rate (bradycardia)
Comments:	not suitable if sensitive to menthol

Other Medicines

Activated charcoal

How taken:	biscuits
Availability:	over the counter
Action:	neutralizes stomach acids and intestinal gas and alleviates bloating, distension and excess wind
Possible side-effects:	none reported

Activated dimeticone/ simethicone

How taken:	liquid, compound
Availability:	over the counter
Action:	coats stomach acids to alleviate colicky pain and wind
Possible side-effects:	none reported

Paracetamol

How taken:	tablets, liquid, compound
Availability:	over the counter and prescription
Action:	thought to act at spinal cord and brain to block 'pain pathways'
Possible side-effects:	rarely - acute pancreatitis, blood disorders, rashes
Comments:	risk of overdose so follow label instructions; avoid compound preparations containing caffeine, which may aggravate symptoms

Ondansetron (seratonergic antagonist)

How taken:	tablets, liquid, suppositories
Availability:	prescription only
Action:	acts at 5-HT3 receptor sites to reduce bowel movement and alleviate diarrhoea, abdominal pain and distension
Possible side-effects:	chest pain, constipation, flushing, headache, high blood pressure (hypertension), hypersensitivity, irregular heart rate (arrhythmia), seizures, slow heart rate (bradycardia); suppositories only: rectal irritation

Antidepressants

Citalopram (SSRI)

How taken:	tablets (low dose)
Availability:	prescription only
Action:	reduces visceral hypersensitivity, relaxes bowel, blunts gastrocolonic response, possible anticholinergic actions; alleviates spasms, abdominal pain, bloating, improves general well-being
Possible side-effects:	abdominal pain, amnesia, constipation, diarrhoea, dyspepsia, migraine, nausea, palpitations, skin rashes, visual disturbances and vomiting
Comments:	side-effects less common in the low doses used in IBS

Paroxetine (SSRI)

Taken:	tablets (low dose)
Availability:	prescription only
Action:	reduces visceral hypersensitivity, relaxes bowel, blunts gastrocolonic response, possible anticholinergic actions; alleviates spasms, abdominal pain, bloating, improves general well-being
Possible side-effects:	abdominal pain, amnesia, constipation, diarrhoea, dyspepsia, migraine, nausea, palpitations, skin rashes, visual disturbances and vomiting
Comments:	side-effects less common in low doses used in IBS

Amitriptyline hydrochloride (Tricyclic)

How taken:	tablets (low dose)
Availability:	prescription only
Action:	alleviates general IBS symptoms, improves general well-being
Possible side-effects:	wide range of side-effects reported, including blurred vision, constipation, dry mouth, irregular heart beat, nausea, sedation, sweating, skin rashes and weight gain
Comments:	side-effects less common in low doses used in IBS

Imipramine hydrochloride (Tricyclic)

How taken:	tablets (low dose)
Availability:	prescription only
Action:	alleviates general IBS symptoms, improves general well-being
Possible side-effects:	blurred vision, constipation, dry mouth, irregular heart beat, nausea, sedation, sweating, skin rashes and weight gain
Comments:	side-effects less common in the low doses used in IBS

Nortriptyline (Tricyclic)

How taken:	tablets (low dose)
Availability:	prescription only
Action:	alleviates general IBS symptoms, improves general well-being
Possible side-effects:	wide range of side-effects reported, including blurred vision, constipation, dry mouth, irregular heart beat, nausea, sedation, sweating, skin rashes and weight gain
Comments:	side-effects less common in low doses used in IBS; nortriptyline less sedating than amitriptyline hydrochloride

Trimipramine (Tricyclic)

How taken:	tablets, capsules
Availability:	prescription only
Action:	alleviates general IBS symptoms, improves general well-being
Possible side-effects:	blurred vision, constipation, dry mouth, irregular heart beat, nausea, sedation, sweating, skin rashes and weight gain
Comments:	side-effects less common in the low doses used in IBS

Sedatives

Buspirone hydrochloride

How taken:	tablets
Availability:	prescription only
Action:	reduces anxiety and stress, helps alleviate diarrhoea and rectal urgency, improves general well-being
Possible side-effects:	nausea, dizziness, headache, lightheadedness, nervousness; (less common) rapid heart rate (tachycardia), palpitations, chest pain, dry mouth, fatigue and sweating
Comments:	short-term use only, except under specialist care

Diazepam

How taken:	tablets
Availability:	prescription only
Action:	reduces anxiety
Possible side-effects:	drowsiness, lightheadedness; (less common) headaches, vertigo, high blood pressure, gastrointestinal disturbances, visual disturbances

Chapter Eleven

Psychological Treatment

Anxiety states, panic disorders and depressive illness are more common among IBS sufferers than non-sufferers. There are also close links between IBS and 'psychosocial' factors such as relationship difficulties, bereavement and trauma. Such factors have a major influence not only on the frequency and severity of symptoms, but also on patients' overall health, the frequency of visits to the doctor, and the success or otherwise of treatment. Therefore, dealing with psychosocial and psychological issues will have an important bearing on symptoms and on the success of any treatment programme.

Just talking to a doctor about life problems can help alleviate symptoms such as anxiety and depression, especially when combined with stress-avoidance techniques (see Chapter Eight) and, in some cases, medication (see Chapter Ten). But many sufferers will benefit from a more structured programme of psychological treatment.

Choosing a Therapy

Psychotherapy may be carried out by a counsellor, clinical psychologist, consultant psychiatrist, an analyst or other therapist, depending on the therapy and the nature of the problem. Some therapies bring out deep-seated psychological issues, often involving childhood experiences, past or present relationships, or physical or emotional traumas. Other therapies offer advice and suggestions to help you modify your behaviour or plan 'coping strategies' (practical ways of dealing with your anxieties) to reduce the impact your symptoms are having on your life.

If your problems are related to a partner or other family member, you may be referred to a therapist who specializes in relationship counselling or family therapy. In such cases your partner and/or children will usually be expected to attend as well.

Analytical (or psychodynamic) therapy, cognitive-behavioural therapy (CBT), counselling and hypnotherapy may be helpful for IBS. Other forms of therapy may also be of benefit, including gestalt therapy, humanistic psychology, primal therapy and transactional analysis.

Analytical (Psychodynamic) Therapy

Analytical therapy may be recommended for IBS patients whose symptoms are linked to deep-seated issues arising from traumatic experiences in their past, particularly during childhood, or relationships with family members. The therapy helps you to make connections between such issues and your current harmful or destructive patterns of behaviour. For example, if you felt rejected by an opposite-sex parent you may find it difficult to form satisfactory relationships. You may be so fearful of rejection that you erect unconscious barriers that prevent relationships from becoming more intimate. The conflict between your need for lasting and fulfilling emotional ties and your fear of rejection can cause severe stress and trigger or aggravate your symptoms. By learning to understand such deep-seated problems, you may find it easier to modify your behaviour in a way that allows future relationships to develop normally.

Analytical therapists (or analysts) conduct sessions mainly on a one-to-one basis. Some therapists also organize group sessions made up of people with similar problems, such as co-dependency, jealousy, panic disorder, obsessive-compulsive disorder, and so on.

Cognitive-Behavioural Therapy

As the name suggests, this therapy brings together two approaches - cognitive and behavioural. It is usually conducted by a clinical psychologist, consultant psychiatrist or specially trained nurse. By combining the two approaches, therapists have a wider range of 'tools' at their disposal and so can tailor the treatment to the needs of the individual.

Cognitive therapy is based on the theory that destructive patterns of behaviour often stem from the negative way in which people perceive the world and their part in it (their 'cognitions'). Negative views are self-fulfilling. If you regard yourself as being unattractive, unintelligent, uninteresting, etc., others can come to see you in the same light. Their low opinion reinforces your poor view of yourself, and you become trapped in a vicious circle.

In psychometric studies, IBS patients commonly believe they have little control over their lives or what happens to them (in psychological tests this is called your 'external locus of control'). They feel that everything bad that happens to them is their fault, while good things happen purely by chance. Other patients have unrealistic expectations of their abilities: either their expectations are too high, in which case they despise themselves for failing, or too low, in which case they are reluctant to try anything new or ambitious for fear the attempt will end in disaster. Negative or destructive attitudes like these can have a direct influence on your self-image, and hence your emotional state, behaviour and IBS symptoms.

Cognitive therapy aims to correct such negative attitudes by boosting your confidence and self-esteem. The therapist encourages you to see yourself, and the events that affect you, in a better light and teaches you to react to other people more positively. When you find that others now respond to you more favourably, it reinforces your good view of yourself and proves to you that you are worthy of being liked and appreciated.

Behavioural therapy aims to help you to recognize and modify destructive patterns of behaviour. The approach is based on the theory that such behaviour patterns are learned, through repeated bad experiences - a form of negative reinforcement. If behaviour has been learned, it follows from this that it can be unlearned, by replacing bad experiences with good ones and by using positive reinforcement.

For example, some IBS patients suffer from faecal urgency - the feeling that when the urge to go to the toilet comes on they will not be able to hold on. This may have come about because of previous experience, such as being in a public place and needing desperately to go to the toilet when no toilet was available. This causes feelings of fear and panic. If the experience is repeated or has embarrassing consequences, such as incontinence, patients learn to associate being away from home with fear and panic, and feel safe and relaxed only when indoors.

In severe cases, patients' fear of the outdoors and the need to be always in range of a toilet can severely restrict their lives. This is known as a 'maladaptive' coping strategy. It can lead to a sense of isolation and depression that can exacerbate the symptoms.

The therapist uses various techniques to try to reverse this behaviour, for example by helping patients feel more relaxed and less panicky when out and about in public. Patients are also taught coping strategies they can use. For example, you might be encouraged to make one scheduled 'toilet stop' on a journey - regardless of whether you need to. You can then complete the journey with confidence, knowing you will not need to go again.

Other IBS sufferers may visit the toilet, perfectly normally, every morning, but go back four or five times during the day because of a feeling that they have not completely evacuated their bowels. Although this is a false impression, it is no less distressing for that. The therapist helps patients accept that one trip to the toilet is sufficient, in their case, and that they have no need to make additional visits. Once patients overcome the 'compulsion' to keep going back to the toilet, they can relax and ignore these false signals.

Counselling

At its simplest, one-to-one counselling means talking issues through. The counsellor's job is not to instruct, but to help you face up to problems and find a way to deal with them constructively. Counselling is not regarded as an appropriate treatment if you are suffering from a serious psychological or psychiatric disorder, in which case specialist help, provided by a clinical psychologist or consultant psychiatrist, may be more suitable.

IBS sufferers are often surprised to discover that the emotional release of talking about, for example, work or relationship difficulties, or other personal concerns, can have a dramatic effect on IBS. Until they attend counselling sessions, sufferers may find it difficult to accept a connection between their symptoms and other areas of their lives.

During a one-to-one counselling session, the counsellor helps you to discover what lies at the root of your problems and to discover the best way to deal with it. It can help you to gain real insights into your situation and face up to the need to make changes. You may have never looked at things objectively before, or have been denying to yourself that a problem exists.

Group counselling brings together several people with similar problems, so they can discuss the issues facing them, openly, with other group members. In the case of IBS sufferers, group members may be people whose symptoms are exacerbated by, for example, relationship or other personal problems.

Although a trained counsellor is usually present during a group meeting, he or she often lets the group determine how the session will progress. By interacting with other members, clients gain insight into their problems. They are also reassured by knowing there are others in a similar situation.

Hypnotherapy

At one time, hypnotherapy was mainly a tool of analytical therapy, to help patients reveal past traumas. Now hypnotherapy is increasingly being used in other disciplines, including pain- and stress-management. Doctors - and many lay hypnotherapists - also use hypnosis for conditions such as IBS.

Hypnotherapy induces a deeply relaxed mental condition which makes clients more receptive to suggestions. The hypnotic state is similar to that seen in other self-induced mind states, such as meditation. Hypnosis does not render you unconscious, and you cannot be compelled to act in a way that is alien to your normal behaviour or codes of conduct.

Hypnotherapy adds more psychological 'weight' to conscious actions of free will, such as keeping to a diet or giving up smoking. Remarkably, the hypnotic state can also bypass the conscious mind and tap into those systems that regulate automatic processes - ones which, normally, you have no direct control over. Subjects are then able, for example, to lower their blood pressure when under stress, or raise their pain threshold, even to the point where they can undergo surgery or dental treatment without an anaesthetic.

Hypnotherapy has been used for selected IBS patients for many years. It can act indirectly - by aiding stress-management, for example - or work directly by alleviating bowel symptoms such as pain and bloating, and improving bowel function. This targeted technique is known as 'gut-directed hypnotherapy'.

Although it is not certain how the technique improves symptoms, it may act via the sympathetic nervous system to reduce or inhibit nerve signals emanating from the bowel, and so moderate bowel activity.

Your doctor may perform hypnotherapy, or may refer you to a specialist who offers this service. Alternatively, you could ask your doctor to recommend a lay therapist who has helped IBS sufferers in the past.

At your first session with the hypnotherapist, you may be asked about your medical and family history and about the exact nature of your symptoms. This enables the therapist to tailor the treatment to your specific needs.

Hypnotherapists have various ways of inducing hypnosis. They may speak softly and soothingly, while asking you to look at a light or at an object at the edge of your vision. You are then given suggestions to ease your symptoms. For example, abdominal pain may be likened to noise from a badly tuned radio set. By turning down the volume control you reduce the level of pain. You may be taught self-hypnosis techniques to manage your symptoms while at home or at work. Some people find it helps to use a self-hypnosis audio tape in order to enter the hypnotic state.

Gestalt Therapy

This form of treatment is based on the theory that inhibitions formed in childhood stop you from responding fully and openly to situations in adulthood. Perhaps you have been taught to 'hold back' in order to conform to your parents' standards of behaviour. This can cause conflict between your internal desires and your external actions, leading to distorted behaviour patterns that can only be resolved by discovering your true self.

The therapist helps you to view your life more clearly and objectively, to value yourself and to understand what you want out of life. Gestalt therapists use various techniques to enable you to resolve internal conflicts. You may work in groups, pairs, or one-to-one with the therapist, and express yourself through, for example, art or dance. Subjects are often encouraged to 'act out' a relationship with another person by, for example, playing both parts in an imagined discussion with a partner or relative.

Humanistic Psychology

Humanistic psychology is similar to gestalt therapy. It is based on the theory that behaviour as an adult stems from learned behaviour in childhood - in particular the belief that your actions are not determined by yourself (and so are not true examples of free will), but follow certain guidelines or pre-conditions set by parents and other adults.

This therapy rejects any approach, including analysis, which encourages a 'victim mentality'. Instead, the therapist aims to bolster your belief in yourself and to reduce your dependence on others. The approach is closer to counselling than to psychotherapy, in that the therapist guides you to reach an understanding of your situation unprompted. You are encouraged to contrast how you appear to yourself with how you appear to others. You can then compare how you behave in the real world with how you would like to behave. By this means, you uncover your true nature and desires, and discover how to achieve what you truly want.

Primal Therapy

This therapy is based on the theory that psychological difficulties in adulthood arise from suppressed childhood feelings of hurt and anger, especially those resulting from lack of parental affection or frequent abuse. Only by expressing these feelings in an intense outpouring of emotion - the 'primal scream' - can adults come to terms with the hurt inside them and begin to live normal lives.

Primal therapy is an intensive psychological treatment, lasting several hours and usually carried out at weekends. It can be highly traumatic and so is not without its risks, but many people feel that it has had a dramatic impact on their lives.

Transactional Analysis (TA)

This form of therapy aims to help you to develop a mature and realistic attitude towards life - particularly in regard to relationships with others -

rather than coming to any deeper understanding about your true self.

TA incorporates different aspects of several approaches, including Freudian analytical therapy, cognitive-behavioural therapy and humanistic psychology. It focuses mainly on one aspect - interchanges (or 'transactions') with other people - and so is regarded as a quick and practical way of tackling relationship difficulties resulting from problem behaviour patterns.

According to TA theory, there are three sides to your personality: the 'parent', which forms the attitudes, judgements and values you have developed through the influence of parents and teachers; the 'adult', which is your acquired ability to make objective assessments and decisions regarding the world around you; and the 'child', made up of childhood experiences and memories which continue to influence your behaviour as an adult.

The 'child' is sub-divided into the 'natural' child, which is the origin of feelings such as creativity, love, intimacy, joy, play and security, and the 'adapted' child, which enables you to relate to others (either positively, by participating in groups, or negatively, by being withdrawn and rebellious). Relationship problems are believed to arise from the unconscious expression of negative aspects of your 'child' and 'parent' personas. As a result, you start to play damaging 'games' or 'transactions' with others.

In TA, the therapist works in a group setting so that patients learn collectively how the different facets of their personality interact, and so form more constructive 'transactions' with others.

Other Therapies

There are many specialized types of psychotherapy, and it is not possible to feature them all here. It is best to choose one that has been recommended by a doctor or other relevant health professional. Reputable psychotherapies have a recognized governing body which can put you in touch with an accredited therapist in your area.

Case Study: John
The specialist in charge of John's case decided to refer him to a clinical psychologist: 'She was really good. She gave me the confidence that although I knew all the toilets on my journey, I only needed to use them about once or twice a week, at 'hotspots', as she called them. We narrowed it down so that I made one planned stop, at a petrol station, say, roughly halfway along my journey. I'd go to the toilet there and know I could finish the journey without stopping. I often didn't really need to go, but that didn't matter. Having made that one stop I knew I would be OK. That has made a big difference to my life.'

ChapterTwelve

ComplementaryTherapies and IBS

There are several complementary therapies which may be of benefit in the treatment and/or management of IBS, either directly by relieving pain and other symptoms, or indirectly by aiding relaxation and alleviating stress.

Always seek an accredited, experienced and fully trained therapist. All the established therapies have their own governing body which can supply a list of accredited therapists based in your area. It is also wise to tell your doctor that you are receiving complementary treatment, to ensure the therapy does not conflict with any treatment he or she has prescribed.

Aromatherapy

The link between aroma and mood is well known. There are strong nerve connections between the olfactory (sense of smell) regions of the brain and the limbic system, the brain's emotional centre. Aromatherapy involves the use of a range of therapeutic oils, known as 'essential oils', derived mainly from plants. These oils may be inhaled from a special oil burner, or diluted with a carrier oil such as sweet almond and massaged into the body, where they are absorbed through the skin. By adding a few drops to a bath, you both inhale and absorb these oils - as well as benefiting from the therapeutic effect of the warm water.

Massage, with or without oils, can ease abdominal pain, aid relaxation, ease stress and enhance emotional and physical well-being. Using aromatic oils may enhance this effect. Aromatherapy massage works best when performed by a trained therapist, but it can be beneficial when given by a friend, partner, or even when self-administered. Massaging the abdomen relieves abdominal tension, improves bowel function and aids digestion. Massaging areas of tension in your body, such as your face, neck, shoulders and legs, may relieve stress.

Self-massage forAbdominal Pain

The following self-massage can be performed sitting, standing or lying down. You can do it without essential oils if you prefer, using talc instead. For an aromatherapy massage, mix 3 drops each of essential oil of peppermint and black pepper with 20 ml (4 tsp) of sweet almond oil or other carrier oil (most nut or seed oils are suitable for massage - but avoid if you have a nut allergy). You can also buy ready-prepared massage oils.

Dip the fingers of one hand into your oil mixture and rest them on your abdomen, just under your breastbone. Place your other hand over the first and use both hands together to knead the oil into the skin, using a gentle clockwise movement.

There are other essential oils you can try to alleviate IBS symptoms, relieve stress and aid relaxation, including German and Roman chamomile, hops, lavender, melissa, neroli, rose otto, slippery elm and sweet marjoram. They can be used in an oil burner, sprinkled over pot pourri, mixed with a carrier oil and massaged into the skin, or you can add some to a bath.

You could try different oils and experiment with various combinations to discover which ones are most effective for you. As a rule, though, essential oils work best when used individually. Avoid mixing more than two or three oils, or the effect can be overpowering.

Caution
Essential oils are highly concentrated, so never take them internally, and never apply them undiluted to your skin. If you have sensitive skin, test first by mixing a few drops of essential oil with a carrier oil and apply a little to your arm. Leave for a while and check for any reaction. If you are pregnant, ask an accredited aromatherapist to recommend 'safe' essential oils. There is little evidence to suggest that, in the tiny amounts normally used, essential oils can harm mother or baby when applied externally. However, as a precaution, it may be best to avoid direct skin contact (for example, in a massage or bath).

Homoeopathy
Homoeopathy, developed in the 19th century by the German physician Samuel Hahneman, is based on two rather controversial beliefs: that substances which trigger symptoms of a particular illness (when consumed at full strength by a healthy person) can heal a person who is suffering from that illness (if taken in dilute form), and that the more a homoeopathic medicine is diluted, the more powerful it becomes. In fact, homoeopathic remedies are so dilute that the active ingredient can't be detected in scientific tests. Homoeopathic medicines are extracted from various plant, animal and mineral sources. The extract is then diluted a set number of times - a process known as 'potentization'. The number given after the name of the remedy - aloe 6c, for example - indicates the number of times it has been diluted, and hence its potency.

During a homoeopathic consultation, the therapist will ask you about your general health, lifestyle and medical history. He or she will seek to find out about all your symptoms and what influences their appearance, frequency and severity. The therapist will then prescribe a highly individualized remedy based on an appraisal of your health, temperament and symptoms.

Although a personal consultation is more effective than self-treatment, it is possible to buy homoeopathic remedies from health shops and pharmacies. These are not as dilute (nor as powerful) as a therapist would prescribe.

The following homoeopathy remedies may be recommended for IBS:

Aloe 6c	*for diarrhoea accompanied by burning rectal pain*
Argentum nit. 6	*for alternating IBS with colicky pain and flatulence*
Arsenicum album 6c	*for diarrhoea accompanied by abdominal pain, anxiety, restlessness and chill*
Colocynthis 6 or 30	*for griping abdominal pain*
Colchicum 6	*for diarrhoea, abdominal pain and nausea*
China 6c	*for diarrhoea with flatulence*
Nux vomica 6c	*for intestinal spasms and constipation*
Podophyllum 6c	*for diarrhoea with early morning abdominal cramps.*

European Herbalism

Traditional European herbalism now includes herbs from many parts of the world, especially North America. The remedies are most effective when administered by an experienced medical herbalist. However, herbal remedies are available from health stores or you can prepare your own, which has the additional advantage of being a useful distraction, helping to take your mind off your symptoms.

Many herbs recommended for IBS act directly on the bowel wall to alleviate muscle spasms and cramping, and to promote regular bowel movement. They may also relax the muscles of the digestive tract to release trapped wind and relieve bloating, flatulence and indigestion. Some herbs contain substances such as pectin and mucilage, which soothe the digestive tract. Others have a calming and mood-enhancing action, and so act indirectly by easing stress, anxiety and depression.

Preparations

Herbal remedies are usually taken in an *infusion*. This is a drink made like tea, by putting the chopped flowers, leaves or seeds into a tea pot, pouring boiling water over them, and leaving to steep for 5-10 minutes. You then strain the mixture into a cup, add sugar or honey to taste and leave to cool a little before drinking.

Some herbs may be effective in combination. For example, you can make an infusion using a mixture of 1 tsp each of agrimony, chamomile and lemon balm.

Another method, suitable for tough plant material, such as bark, is in a *decoction*. Here the herbal extract is added to boiling water and simmered for 15 minutes to extract the active ingredients. Again, add sugar or honey to taste and leave to cool. You can drink three or four cups a day.

Caution
Always consult an accredited, qualified and experienced medical herbalist before taking herbal medicines. Obtain herbs and herbal remedies from established suppliers only. Never use fresh herbs (especially wild plants) unless you can make a positive identification. If you are pregnant, or suffering from high blood pressure, heart, kidney or liver disease, or other serious disorder, always check with your doctor first.

Here are some examples of herbs that can help to ease IBS symptoms:

agrimony
(Agrimonia eupatoria) *contains astringents which are said to have a 'drying' action on the bowel, and so may alleviate diarrhoea*
infusion: *add 1 tsp of dried leaves to 300 mls (^{1}/2 pt) of boiling water and steep for 10 minutes*

catmint or catnip
(Nepeta cataria) *alleviates bloating, spasms, cramping, flatulence and indigestion, and promotes regular bowel movement*
infusion: *add 1 tsp of dried leaves to 300 mls (^{1}/2 pt) of boiling water and steep for 10 minutes*

chamomile
(Matricaria recutita) *soothes the bowel and alleviates muscle spasms, helping to prevent pain, diarrhoea or constipation and release trapped wind (also said to calm nerves and aid restful sleep)*
infusion: *add 1 tsp of dried flowers to 300 mls (^{1}/2 pt) of boiling water and steep for 10 minutes*

dill
(Anethum graveolens) *eases spasms, bloating and flatulence*
decoction: *add 1 tbsp whole fennel seeds to 300 mls (^{1}/2 pt) of water in a small saucepan, bring to the boil and simmer for 10 minutes*

fennel
(Foeniculum vulgare)   alleviates spasms, bloating and flatulence
infusion: add 1 tsp of crushed seeds to 300 mls (^{1}/2 pt) of boiling water and steep for 15 minutes
decoction: add 2 tsp whole fennel seeds to 300 mls (^{1}/2 pt) of water in a saucepan, bring to the boil and simmer for 5 minutes

ginger
(Zingiber officinale)   relieves spasms and dyspepsia and assists the action of other herbal remedies
infusion: add 1 tsp of chopped ginger root to 300 mls (^{1}/2 pt) of boiling water and steep for 10 minutes

lemon balm
(Melissa angustifolia)   alleviates bloating, spasms, cramping, flatulence and indigestion and promotes regular bowel movement
infusion: add 1-2 tsp of dried herb to 300 mls (^{1}/2 pt) of boiling water and steep for 10 minutes

peppermint
(Mentha X piperita)   alleviates bloating, spasms, cramping, flatulence and indigestion and promotes regular bowel movement
infusion: add 1 tsp (heaped) of dried, chopped peppermint leaves to 250 mls (^{1}/2 pt) of boiling water and steep for 10 minutes; (peppermint oil is also available)

Traditional Chinese Medicine (TCM)

This ancient form of healing takes a multi-disciplinary approach, offering dietary and lifestyle advice as well as various integrated therapies such as acupuncture, herbalism and massage. TCM is based on the belief that there are two fundamental yet opposing forces of nature - *yin* and *yang*.

Therapists aim to identify and correct imbalances in these two forces, and so restore harmony and health to the body. The two therapies receiving most interest in the West are Chinese herbal medicine and acupuncture.

Chinese Herbal Medicine

This therapy worries some Western doctors, mainly because Chinese herbal remedies can contain mixtures of 20 or more plant extracts, often in non-standardized formulations. This makes them difficult to evaluate scientifically, and increases the risk of adulteration with toxic substances. Some patients have needed hospital treatment (including major surgery) after taking contaminated herbs.

Nevertheless, many IBS sufferers swear by Chinese medicines. Researchers who tested five Chinese herbal extracts reported that patients showed significant improvement in their abdominal pain and other symptoms, compared with a placebo.

Chinese herbalists select different combinations of herbs, according to the symptoms and general health of the patient. The two main ingredients in Chinese herbal medicines are the 'emperor' and 'deputy' herbs. Other ingredients, or 'messenger' herbs, are used to moderate the effects of the main herbs. These medicines are normally taken as an infusion. Examples of Chinese herbal mixtures include:

Chinese angelica, rhubarb,	
peach seed and notopterygium root	*to relieve constipation*
liquorice, magnolia bark,	
tangerine peel and white atractylodes	*to treat diarrhoea and bloating.*

Caution
Always consult an accredited, qualified and experienced medical herbalist before taking herbal medicines. If you are pregnant, or suffering from high blood pressure, heart, kidney or liver disease, or other serious disorder, always check with your doctor first.

Acupuncture

Acupuncture involves the application of needles to certain key sites, or 'acupoints', on the body. The acupuncturist seeks to manipulate a form of 'vital energy' called *chi* (or *qi*). *Chi* is said to flow through the body along energy channels called (in English) 'meridians'. Each meridian controls the flow of *chi* to one or more organ or bodily system.

According to TCM philosophy, a blockage in a channel leads to disrupted energy flows, congested *chi*, and an imbalance of *yin* and *yang*. This causes symptoms involving the bodily system served by that meridian. Acupoints are sites where meridians pass close to the surface of the body. By inserting a needle at relevant points on the body, the therapist relieves the blockage, or diverts the energy flow, and allows *chi* to flow freely again.

Some studies suggest that acupuncture might be helpful in IBS. In one trial, a group of IBS patients was treated with acupuncture sessions three times a week for two weeks. In the following four weeks, patients reported significant improvement in abdominal pain and other symptoms, and in their quality of life. Similar results were seen in a comparison group who had relaxation sessions instead. Significantly, though, when patients were interviewed again four weeks later, the acupuncture group reported a continuing reduction in pain. This was not the case in the relaxation group.

If you are interested in trying acupuncture, you should be aware that some trials conducted more recently have not confirmed these results.

In a typical acupuncture consultation, the therapist takes note of all the patient's symptoms, not only those specifically related to IBS. The therapist then carries out a physical examination, manipulating the limbs, taking the pulse, and looking at the tongue and eyes. Tenderness at any acupoint is also noted. Taken together, this information enables the therapist to locate the site of blocked or congested *chi* that is causing the symptoms.

Treatment involves three or more sessions in as many weeks. Needles are placed in appropriate acupoints and a wooden chip may be taped to the ear, at a site that corresponds to one of the key acupoints. Patients return weekly to report their progress and receive further treatment.

The channel responsible for the healthy functioning of the bowel (among other organs) is the hand or *chao yin* meridian. It is also known as the triple energizer (TE). One of the most important acupoints for the treatment of irritable bowel syndrome (and constipation) is *zhigou* or TE6 - in other words, point six on the triple energizer meridian. It is located on the back of the right arm, about three finger-widths above the wrist, between the lower arm bones (radius and ulna). The exact position is determined by the acupuncturist, according to a patient's height and build.

Another key acupoint, for flatulence and bloating, is ST36 (point 36 on the stomach meridian) located four finger-widths below the kneecap (with knee slightly bent), and one finger-width to the side of the shin bone.

Acupressure

You can stimulate acupoints yourself, using *acupressure* - a therapy similar to acupuncture, but using the tip of the middle finger instead of a needle. Acupressure is considered less effective than acupuncture, but is easy to self-administer, requires no equipment, and can be performed wherever you are.

To find the right spot, press your finger all over the TE6 or ST36 area (described above) until you feel a numb, tender or tingling sensation. Apply firm pressure at a 90-degree angle to the skin and maintain for 20 seconds, release for 10 seconds, and reapply for 20 seconds. Keep doing this five or six times. Repeat the process at regular intervals over the next few hours.

This is one of the oldest health care systems in the world. The name is derived from two Ancient Sanskrit words: *ayus* meaning 'life' or 'longevity', and *veda* meaning 'knowledge' or 'science'. Like Traditional Chinese Medicine, the principle of Ayurveda is to achieve harmony of body and spirit by balancing opposing forces, in this case three *doshas* or humours: *vata* (wind), *pitta* (bile) and *kapha* (phlegm).

Ayurveda combines several approaches, including diet, herbalism and massage. But the practice that has been adopted most enthusiastically in the West is yoga. This has practical benefits for the management of IBS.

Yoga

The term *yoga* is a Sanskrit word meaning 'union' and describes the state of calm, physical and mental harmony and spiritual 'oneness' that adepts strive for. Yoga involves deep breathing, meditation, movements and static postures. Many of the relaxation techniques featured elsewhere in this book have been borrowed or adapted from traditional yoga exercises.

Yogic breathing and meditation, in particular, are extremely effective as aids to relaxation, thereby alleviating stress. Yoga has helped people to alleviate heart disorders by reducing their pulse rate and lowering their blood pressure. Some of the postures, when combined with yogic breathing techniques, may aid digestion and alleviate abdominal disorders.

Yoga is thought to be most beneficial, however, when taught as a complete philosophy by an experienced yoga teacher, and practised regularly.

One yoga posture that may be beneficial in the case of IBS is a form of forward bend called *uttanasana*.

Caution

Seek your doctor's advice before attempting this posture if you have high blood pressure or suffer back problems.

1   To start, stand straight with your head, neck and spine in alignment, and your feet slightly apart and parallel. Put your arms by your sides, fingers pointing straight down, and gaze steadily ahead. Take several slow breaths, drawing the air deep down into your abdomen, until you feel relaxed.
2   Breathing in deeply and slowly, lift your arms over your head with your palms facing each other and slightly apart.
3   Breathing out slowly, bend forward at the hips (not the waist) and, with knees slightly bent, reach down and grasp your ankles, letting your head and upper body relax towards the floor. Take several slow, deep breaths to help your upper body relax completely.

4 Slowly straighten up and return to the start position. Continue to breathe slowly and deeply, and feel any remaining tension draining down through the soles of your feet into the floor.

Other Complementary Therapies

The following complementary therapies may be of benefit to IBS sufferers, either by alleviating bowel problems or promoting relaxation and relief from stress and anxiety:

Art therapy	Subjects use painting, drawing or other forms of artistic endeavour to express their deep-rooted anxieties and frustrations and release the pent-up tension that is contributing to their symptoms.
Autogenic training	This relaxation therapy has links with meditation, visualization and self-hypnosis. Subjects are taught six techniques designed to induce calmness by focusing their attention on sensations in separate areas of the body. These sensations are: heartbeat, breathing, coolness of the forehead, heaviness in the neck, shoulders and limbs, and warmth in the limbs and stomach.
Biofeedback	Here, subjects are linked up to a machine that registers, for example, heart rate, blood pressure or electrical resistance on the skin, and readings are displayed on a screen. You use a chosen relaxation technique to, for example, reduce your blood pressure and monitor the display screen to check how well the relaxation technique is working.
Osteopathy	This manipulative therapy involves gentle manual pressure and controlled movement of the joints. The osteopath aims to bring the bones, muscles, ligaments and associated structures of the body back into alignment, and so restore proper functioning to bodily systems.
T'ai-chi ch'uan	This involves carefully arranged sequences of slow, flowing movements combined with breathing and meditation techniques designed to enhance balance, release tension and develop a sense of mental, physical and spiritual harmony.

References

Aggarwal A, Cutts TF, Abell TL *et al.*, 'Predominant symptoms in irritable bowel syndrome correlate with specific autonomic nervous system abnormalities' *Gastroenterology 1994; 106: 945-50*

Agréus L, Svärdsudd K, Nyrén O *et al.*, 'Irritable bowel syndrome and dyspepsia in the general population: overlap and lack of stability over time', *Gastroenterology 1995; 109: 671-80*

Akehurst R, Kaltenthaler E, 'Treatment of irritable bowel syndrome: a review of randomised controlled trials', *Gut 2001; 48: 272-82*

Anon, *Slim & Healthy Cookery (London: Ebury Press, 1989)*

Belville JW *et al.*, 'Influence of age on pain relief from analgesics', *Journal of the American Medical Association 1971; 217: 1835-41*

Bennet EJ et al., 'Level of Chronic life stress predicts clinical outcome in irritable bowel syndrome', *Gut 1998; 43: 256-61*

Bensoussan A, Talley NJ, Hing M *et al.*, 'Treatment of irritable bowel syndrome with Chinese herbal medicine. A randomized controlled trial', *JAMA 1998; 18: 1585-9*

Bueno L, 'New and future drugs in nerve-gut dysfunctions', state-of-the-art lecture. Program and abstracts of the 7th United European Gastroenterology Week; November 13-17, 1999; Rome, Italy

Buts J-P, Bernasconi P, Vaerman J-P *et al.*, 'Stimulation of secretory IgA and secretory component of immunoglobulins in small intestine of rats treated with Saccharomyces boulardii', *Dig Dis Sci. 1990; 35: 251-6*

Cadenas FF, Villanueva A, Iglesias-Canle J *et al.*, 'Clinical course of irritable bowel syndrome (IBS): A 2-3 year follow-up study', program and abstracts of Digestive Disease Week 2001; May 20-23, 2001; Atlanta, Georgia. [Poster #4065]

Camillieri M, Choi MG, 'Review article: irritable bowel syndrome', *Aliment Pharmacol Ther 1997; 11: 3-15*

Chiang CY and Chang CT, 'Peripheral afferent pathway for acupuncture analgesia', *Scientica Sinica 1973; 16 (1): 210-17*

Chokroverty S, *Sleep Disorders Medicine: Basic Science, Technical Considerations and Clinical Aspects (Boston, MA: Butterworth-Heinemann, 1994)*

Christensen J, 'The enteric nervous system', in *An Illustrated Guide to Gastrointestinal Motility (Chichester: John Wiley & Sons, 1998)*

Clouse RE, Prakash C, Anderson RJ *et al.*, 'Antidepressants for functional gastrointestinal symptoms and syndromes: a meta-analysis', program and abstracts of Digestive Disease Week 2001; May 20-23, 2001; Atlanta, Georgia. [Poster #3252]

Collins SM, Valiance B, Barbara G, Borgaonkar M, 'Putative inflammatory and immunological mechanisms in functional bowel disorders', *Baillieres Best Pract Res Clin Gastroenterol* 1999; 13: 429-36

Corney RH, Stanton R, 'Physical symptom severity, psychological and social dysfunction in a series of outpatients with irritable bowel syndrome', *J Psychosom Res* 1990; 34: 483-91

Creed FH, Craig T, Farmer RG, 'Functional abdominal pain, psychiatric illness and life events', *Gut* 1988; 29: 235-42

Dickhaus B, Firooz N, Stain J *et al.*, 'Psychological stress increases visceral sensitivity in patients with irritable bowel syndrome (IBS) but not controls', *Gastroenterology* 2001; 120: A-67

Ellis, N, *Acupuncture in Clinical Practice* (London: Chapman and Hall, 1994)

Elmer GW, McFarland LV, Surawicz CM (eds), *Biotherapeutic agents and infectious diseases* (Totowa, NJ: Humana, 1999)

Elsenbruch S, Harnish MJ, Orr WC, 'Subjective and objective sleep quality in irritable bowel syndrome', *Gastroenterology* 1998; 114: A749

Fass R, Fullerton S, Higa L *et al.*, 'Sleep disturbances in clinic patients with functional bowel disorders', *Am J Gastroenterol* 2000; 95: 1195-1200

Fass R, Fullerton S, Naliboff B *et al.*, 'Sexual dysfunction in patients with irritable bowel syndrome and non-ulcer dyspepsia', *Digestion* 1998; 59: 79-85

Friedlander Y, Kark JD and Stein Y, 'Religious orthodoxy and myocardial infarction in Jerusalem - a case control study', *International Journal of Cardiology* 1986; 10: 33-41

Forbes A, MacAuley S, Chiotakakou-Faliakou E, 'Hypnotherapy and therapeutic audiotape: effective in previously unsuccessfully treated irritable bowel syndrome?', *Int J Colorectal Dis* 2000; 15: 328-34

Francis CY, Whorwell PJ, 'Bran and the irritable bowel syndrome: time for reappraisal', *Lancet* 1994; 344: 39-40

Fry J, Sandler G and Brooks D, *Disease Data Book* (Lancaster: MTP Press, 1986)

Fuller R, 'Probiotics in man and animals', *J Appl Bacteriol* 1989; 66: 365-78

Furness JB, Kunze WA, Bertrand PP, Clerc N, Bornstein JC, 'Intrinsic primary afferent neurons of the intestine', *Prog Neurobiol* 1998; 54: 1-18

Gaynes B, Drossman DA, 'The role of psychosocial factors in irritable bowel syndrome', *Baillieres Clin Gastroenterol* 1999; 13: 437-452

Gershon MD, 'Roles played by 5-hydroxytryptamine in the physiology of the bowel', *Aliment Pharmacol Ther* 1999; 13(suppl 2): 15-30

Guthrie E, Creed F, Dawson G, *et al.*, 'A randomised controlled trial of psychotherapy in patients with refractory irritable bowel syndrome', *Br J Psych* 1993; 163: 315-21

Hammer J, Tally NJ, 'Diagnostic criteria for the irritable bowel syndrome', *Am J Med* 1999; 107: 5S-11S

Han CS, 'Physiological and neurochemical basis of acupuncture in analgesia', in TO Cheng (ed.), *The International Textbook of Cardiology* (New York: Pergamon Press, 1986): 1124-32

Harvey RF, Mauad EC, Brown AM, 'Prognosis in the irritable bowel syndrome: a five-year prospective study', *Lancet* 1987; 1: 963-5

Heaton J, *et al.*, 'Symptoms of irritable bowel syndrome in a British Urban Community: consulters and nonconsulters', *Gastroenterology* 1992; 102: 1962-7

Jackson JL, O'Malley PG, Tomplans G *et al.*, 'Treatment of functional gastrointestinal disorders with anti-depressant medications: a meta-analysis', *Am J Med* 2000; 108: 65-72

Jailwala J, Imperiale TF, Kroenke K, 'Pharmacologic treatment of the irritable bowel syndrome: a systematic review of randomized, controlled trials', *Ann Intern Med* 2000; 133: 136-47

Jarney C and Tindall J, *Acupressure for Common Ailments* (London: Gaia Books, 1991)

Johnsgard KW, *The Exercise Prescription for Depression and Anxiety* (New York: Plenum Press, 1989)

Jones J *et al.*, 'British Society of Gastroenterology Guidelines for the Management of the Irritable Bowel Syndrome', *Gut* 2000: 47 (Suppl 2)

Koloski NA, Talley NJ, Matheson M *et al.*, 'Psychological predictors of irritable bowel syndrome (IBS) and functional dyspepsia (FD) in general population', *Gastroenterology* 2001; 120: A-758

Lembo T, Munakata J, Mertz H *et al.*, 'Evidence for hypersensitivity of lumbar splanchnic afferents in irritable bowel syndrome', *Gastroenterology* 1994; 107: 1686-96

Lu B, Hu Y, Tenner S, 'A randomized controlled trial of acupuncture for irritable bowel syndrome', program and abstracts of the 65th Annual Scientific Meeting of the American College of Gastroenterology; October 16-18, 2000, New York, NY. Poster 268, p. 428

Madisch A, Holtmann G, Sassin I *et al.*, 'Herbal preparations in patients with irritable bowel syndrome: results of a double-blind, randomized, placebo-controlled multicenter trial', *Gastroenterology* 2001: A-134. [Abstract #715]

Malcolm L, *Health Style* (London: Duncan Baird Publishing, 2001)

Mertz H, Naliboff B, Muakat J *et al.*, 'Altered rectal perception is a biological marker of patients with irritable bowel syndrome', *Gastroenterology* 1995; 109: 40-52

Metchnikoff E, *The Prolongation of Life* (G. P. Putnam's Sons, 1908): 161

Morris-Yates A, Talley NJ, Boyce PM, Nandurkar S, Andrews G, 'Evidence of a genetic contribution to functional bowel disorder', *Am J Gastroenterol* 1998; 93: 1311-17

Nanda R *et al.*, 'Food intolerance and the irritable bowel syndrome', *Gut* 1989; 30: 1099-1104

Northcutt AR, Mangel AW, Hamm LR *et al.*, 'Persistent placebo response during a year-long controlled trial of IBS treatment', program and abstracts of Digestive Disease Week 2001; May 20-23, 2001; Atlanta, Georgia. [Poster #3243]

Pert A *et al.*, 'Mechanisms of opiate analgesia and the role of endorphins in pain suppression', in *Advances in Neurology* (vol. 33; New York: Raven Press, 1982): 107-22

Polunin M, *Healing Foods* (London: Dorling Kindersley, 1997)

Poynard T, Regimbeau C, Benhamou Y, 'Meta-analysis of smooth muscle relaxants in the treatment of irritable bowel syndrome', *Aliment Pharmacol Ther* 2001; 15: 355-61

Ramsey DJ and Booth DA (eds), *Thirst: Physiological and Psychological Aspects* (London: Springer-Verlag, 1991)

Rodriguez LAG and Ruigomez A, 'Increased risk of irritable bowel syndrome after bacterial gastroenteritis: cohort study', *BMJ* 1999; 318: 565-6

Sanders KM, Ordog T, Koh SD, Torihashi S, Ward SM, 'Development and plasticity of interstitial cells of Cajal', *Neurogastroenterology & Motility* 1999; 11: 311-38

Sanger GJ, 'Hypersensitivity and hyperreactivity in the irritable bowel syndrome: an opportunity for drug discovery', *Dig Dis* 1999; 17: 90-9

SatioYA, Locke GR, William DE *et al.*, 'The role of psychological distress on symptoms and health care utilization in patients with irritable bowel syndrome', *Gastroenterology* 2000; 118: A399.

Scarpignato C, 'Management of irritable bowel syndrome: novel approaches to the pharmacology of gut motility', *Can J Gastroenterol* 1999; 13: 50A-65A

Serpell JM, 'Beneficial effects of pet ownership on some aspects of human health and behaviour', *Journal of the Royal Society of Medicine* 1991; 84: 717-20

Silk DB, 'Patients' views on IBS', *Int J Gastroenterology* 1998; 3: 20-22

Simren M, Axeisson J, Abrahamsson H, Svediund J, Bjsrnsson ES, 'Symptoms of irritable bowel syndrome in inflammatory bowel disease in remission and relationship to psychological factors', program and abstracts of Digestive Disease Week; May 21-24, 2000; San Diego, California; Abstract 3842

Svendsen JH, Munck LK, Anderson JR, 'Irritable bowel syndrome: prognosis and diagnostic safety. A 5-year follow-up study', *Scand J Gastroenterol* 1985; 20: 415-18

Talley NJ *et al.*, 'Epidemiology of colonic symptoms and the irritable bowel syndrome', *Gastroenterology* 1991; 101: 927-34

Thornley JP, Brough J, Wright T, Neal KR, Jenkins D, Spiller RC, 'Bacterial toxins influence long term bowel dysfunction following Campylobacter enteritis', program and abstracts of Digestive Disease Week; May 21-24, 2000; San Diego, California; Abstract 3841

Tornblom H, Lindberg G, Nyberg B, Veress B, 'Histopathological findings in jejunum of patients with severe irritable bowel syndrome', program and abstracts of Digestive Disease Week; May 21-24, 2000; San Diego, California; Abstract 3840

Tyler VE, 'Product definition deficiencies in clinical studies of herbal medicines', *Scientific Review of Alt Med* 2000; 4(2): 17-21

Van Ginkel R, Voskuijl WP, Benninga MA, Taminiau JAJM, Boeckxstaens GE, 'Do changes in visceral sensation and motility play a role in the pathophysiology of childhood irritable bowel syndrome (IBS)?', *Gastroenterology* 2001; 120: 31-8

Vanderwinden JM, 'Role of interstitial cells of Cajal and their relationship with the enteric nervous system', *Eur J Morphol* 1999; 37: 250-6

Whitehead WE, Crowell MD, Robinson JC *et al.*, 'Effects of stressful life events on bowel symptoms: subjects with irritable bowel syndrome compared to subjects without bowel dysfunction', *Gut* 1992; 33: 825-30

Wood JD, 'Physiology of the enteric nervous system', in LR Johnson (ed), *Physiology of the Gastrointestinal Tract* (New York: Raven, 1994): 423-82

Index

125

Notes